Minor Illness
or Major Disease?

Minor Illness or Major Disease?

Responding to symptoms in the pharmacy

THIRD EDITION

Clive Edwards
BPharm, PhD, MRPharmS
Prescribing Adviser
Tyne & Wear, UK

Paul Stillman
MB, ChB, DRCOG
General Practitioner, Sussex, UK

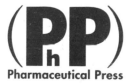

Pharmaceutical Press

Published by the Pharmaceutical Press
1 Lambeth High Street, London SE1 7JN, UK

First edition published 1982
Second edition published 1995
Reprinted 1995, 1997
Third edition published 2000

© Pharmaceutical Press 1982, 1995, 2000

Text design by Barker/Hilsdon, Lyme Regis, Dorset
Typeset by J&L Composition Ltd, Filey, North Yorkshire
Printed in Italy by Rotolito Lombardo SpA

ISBN 0 85369 447 8

A catalogue record for this book is available from the British
Library.

To Pat and Joy

Contents

Preface

Between February 1979 and May 1981, a series of articles was published in *The Pharmaceutical Journal* entitled 'Minor Illness or Major Disease?' It coincided with a period of renewed interest in responding to symptoms by pharmacists, and the articles were collated and published as a book by the Pharmaceutical Press in 1982. The articles were unique at that time because they were written jointly by a pharmacist and a general medical practitioner. This type of joint authorship turned out to be a successful formula and we are delighted to see that other pharmacist authors, writing about the same subject, have also teamed up with medical colleagues. This emphasises that responding to symptoms should be a joint venture between the medical and pharmacy professions and that doctors and pharmacists can work together for the common good of the patient.

Since the original series, responding to symptoms has become a core part of the pharmacy undergraduate curriculum as well as continuing education. Words such as 'diagnosis', which were forbidden in our first series, have now become more acceptable, albeit as a basic screening tool to enable possible serious illness to be referred for a medical opinion and minor self-limiting conditions to be treated with over-the-counter medicines as appropriate. Deregulation of medicines from the prescription-only category to pharmacy medicines continues to provide the pharmacist with a greater armamentarium of medicines for the treatment of minor disorders. Between April 1993 and June 1994 we published a second series of articles in the Journal and this formed the basis of the second edition of the book which was published in 1995.

The demand for advice over the counter in the pharmacy and the desire for patients to self-medicate increases globally on a daily basis. The infrastructure of primary health care in the UK is also changing to meet the needs of patients, with new important roles for nurse practitioners and recommendations for other professionals, besides doctors, to take on the role of prescriber. These changes will alter the way in which patients receive their care, especially for chronic disease and for minor ailments. The role of the community pharmacist remains pivotal in health care, especially with regard to advice for and treatment of minor illness. We are therefore delighted to have had the opportunity to revise *Minor Illness or Major Disease?* and produce the third edition, again in a format that we hope is both easy to read and easy to understand for students and practising professionals.

This third edition contains new illustrations and photographs. Each chapter contains a summary of signs and symptoms that require referral to a doctor and case studies taken from real situations experienced by the authors, which illustrate the application of the text material to pharmacy practice. The title of our original series has been retained, not only for sentimental reasons, but also because it reflects the principal decision which the pharmacist must make after questioning the patient before deciding whether to recommend a course of medication or provide appropriate advice.

Clive Edwards
Paul Stillman
2000

Acknowledgements

We would like to dedicate this book to the staff of *The Pharmaceutical Journal* and to the many colleagues and students who have shown an interest in responding to symptoms over the years.

In particular, we are indebted to Robert Blyth who, as editor of the Journal in 1979, gave us the encouragement to write a series on responding to symptoms under the title 'Minor Illness or Major Disease?' and the medium in which to publish it. This series was reprinted by the Pharmaceutical Press as the first edition of the book. In turn his successor, Douglas Simpson, also encouraged us to go into print again with a second series in the Journal. The final quality of our efforts would not have been the same without the invaluable editorial expertise of Joanna Lumb, senior assistant editor of *The Pharmaceutical Journal*, who steered us through both series in the Journal which formed the core of all three editions of the book. Our thanks also go to the staff of the Pharmaceutical Press over the years and especially to Linda Horrell and Paul Weller for their valuable guidance with this edition.

We would also like to record our friendship with Bernard Hardisty. At the time of our first series, Bernard was employed by an OTC drug manufacturer and he and his company did much to motivate community pharmacists to take seriously their role in responding to symptoms.

We are grateful to Professor Robin Seymour, professor of restorative dentistry at the University of Newcastle, for contributing the chapter on oral and dental disorders, and to Mrs E J Franklin, district chief chiropodist, Mid Downs Health Authority, West Sussex, for advice on the chapter on foot disorders.

Our thanks also to the following for photographs: Science Photo Library; GlaxoWellcome; Wellcome Trust Medical Photographic Library; Medical Slide Library; and the Department of Dermatology, Royal Victoria Infirmary, Newcastle upon Tyne.

About the authors

Clive Edwards studied pharmacy at the School of Pharmacy, London University. He obtained a PhD in pharmacology and has wide experience of community, hospital and academic pharmacy. From 1978 until 1997 he held lectureships and senior lectureships in clinical pharmacy at the Universities of Aston and Newcastle, respectively. He has a wide working knowledge of clinical therapeutics in hospitals and still works as an occasional locum in community pharmacy. He is currently prescribing adviser for a primary care group.

Paul Stillman studied medicine at the University of Bristol, and after vocational training became a principal in general practice in Sussex, where he has remained for 25 years and is now senior partner. He has had a long interest in medical education, and is a course organiser and trainer for general practice. He is also extensively involved in the public awareness of health and illness, and has worked to promote this through television, radio and the press.

1

Introduction

Pharmacists have advised members of the public about the treatment of minor illnesses for as long as the profession has existed. Before embarking on any form of advice or treatment, some initial diagnosis is necessary to exclude any potentially serious cause which may require a medical consultation. This diagnosis of exclusion is one which pharmacists should be able to make in the vast majority of cases that they see every day. It may be thought of as a screening or sieving process which can be achieved by careful, intelligent questioning of the patient. It is a process which many patients take it upon themselves to perform before self-medicating and, generally, they are very competent at it. It is also commonly the *modus operandi* for doctors when a patient presents with symptoms for the first time in general practice.

Clearly, this sort of diagnosis can take on various degrees of sophistication and there is a suitable level at which the pharmacist can participate in the process. At this level it is not difficult, and with a structured approach to questioning, which closely follows that taught to doctors, pharmacists can make valuable judgments as to whether to refer a patient to a doctor or to recommend self-treatment.

The suggested format which follows is one approach that can be used to elicit a comprehensive history.

General rules

Almost too obvious to mention, but crucially important, is the question of who is the patient. Is it the person relating the story or is he/she a representative of the patient? It is difficult to obtain a satisfactory history from a third party. If the patient is not present, it is useful to establish whether the reason for their absence is the severity of symptoms. Parents of young children will give good histories of a child's illness; if the child is present, the severity of the illness and other signs can be observed. In the absence of the patient, pharmacists should reassure themselves that they are in no doubt as to the severity and nature of the disease. If there is any uncertainty, it is unwise to recommend self-treatment.

The patient should first be allowed to explain the illness in his/her own words as a response to a general question such as 'What is the problem?' or 'How do you feel?' This allows the patient to relax and encourages him/her to talk and provide clues that can be followed up by more specific questions later. During this phase of the interview, the pharmacist can observe the demeanour or the attitude of the patient so that the pharmacist can consider the question 'Does the patient look ill?' Some patients can articulate the severity of their illness adequately, but in others non-verbal signs (such as body language) must be observed to distinguish a very sick person from a relatively healthy one. This is particularly relevant in babies, who can indicate their discomfort by refusing to eat, by crying or screaming (even after being picked up) or by being irritable or behaving in some abnormal fashion.

The patient should be asked about current or recent medicines that have been taken, both prescribed (and therefore often for other conditions) and over-the-counter (OTC) (for this illness and for other problems). This is helpful for eliciting any drug-induced symptoms, as well as for establishing whether the patient has already tried a remedy for the present complaint. At some point in the questioning, perhaps later in the more

Table 1.1	A reminder of questions to ask
S	Site or location
I	Intensity or severity
T	Type or nature
D	Duration
O	Onset
W	With (other symptoms)
N	aNnoyed or aggravated by
S	Spread or radiation
I	Incidence or frequency pattern
R	Relieved by

specific questions, any relevant past history can be inquired after, such as personal or family history, together with occupation and social habits, for example smoking, drinking and exercise.

The description of the illness can be expanded by asking more specific and structured questions, which can be prompted by a mnemonic (Table 1.1).

Questions to ask

Site or location

This question can be helpful in diagnosis in some instances, for example where pain is the main symptom. For instance, a pain in the abdomen could be caused by appendicitis (central pain, moving to the right iliac fossa), renal colic (pain in right or left loin or iliac fossa), peptic ulcer (central or epigastric) or biliary colic (right hypochondrium). Similarly, headaches can be unilateral (migraine), frontal (migraine, sinusitis or tension) or occipital (tension, muscle spasm or subarachnoid haemorrhage). The site of a skin rash can distinguish a localised reaction, for example to a watchstrap, from the allergy to an antibiotic in which the whole body may be involved.

Intensity or severity

The intensity or severity of a symptom, such as pain, a skin rash or bleeding from a wound, gives information not only about the likely diagnosis but also about the urgency of a situation. This is essential when considering whether to temporise and monitor the course of a symptom or illness for a little longer, give an OTC medicine or recommend referral to the patient's doctor.

Type or nature

Further description of a symptom can help to differentiate certain conditions. For example, an abdominal pain which is cramp-like or colicky indicates involvement of a hollow organ, such as the bowel or ureter, which contracts due to spasm of smooth muscle in the organ wall. On the other hand, patients often describe the pain of a peptic ulcer as a 'gnawing' pain. Similarly, the appearance of a rash as flat or raised, single or multiple, or blistering or dry lesions can help to differentiate various skin conditions.

Duration

The duration of any symptom must always be established. This information can be helpful to distinguish, say, the headache of migraine (which usually lasts no more than a few hours) from a tension headache (which may persist for several days or weeks). The duration will also help the pharmacist to decide whether to refer in certain situations. For example, a baby who has suffered from diarrhoea for three days requires referral for a medical assessment whereas a baby with diarrhoea of only a few hours' duration may respond adequately to hydration with simple electrolyte mixtures.

Onset

The history of onset of a symptom or illness can provide clues to its likely cause. Thus, abdominal pain and diarrhoea which starts soon after overindulgence in a restaurant or headache which occurs on awakening after an alcoholic binge are likely to require little more than reassurance, sympathy and simple OTC measures.

Accompanying symptoms

Concomitant symptoms may not always be volunteered by the patient, especially if they feel that they are not important or not related to the main symptom about which they are complaining. Such information is, however, crucial to differentiate many disorders. For example, someone who complains of a productive cough or of diarrhoea should be asked if there is blood in the sputum or motions to distinguish between potentially serious disease or more trivial illness. Someone with a red eye that is itching and watery may have a simple allergy while a red eye that is painful or accompanied by some disturbance of vision will require immediate medical attention.

Thus, any symptom should be submitted to a systematic review, inquiring first about other symptomatology within the same body system and then, either by direct questioning or more general open questions (depending on the problem), about any symptoms in other systems.

Factors that aggravate the condition

Although not always relevant, there are some conditions for which inquiry about any factors that worsen the symptom can be valuable. The pain of a peptic ulcer, for example, can be worsened by a heavy meal or alternatively by fasting, while that caused by gallstones will be particularly exacerbated by a fatty meal.

Headaches associated with a raised intracranial pressure will be worse after lying down and therefore worse in the mornings, whereas tension headaches may be better in the mornings but worsen as the day goes on.

Spread or radiation

There are several examples of where a sensation, usually pain, spreads characteristically and almost predictably to another part of the body. In the case of pain, this is known as referred pain. The diagnosis of appendicitis is classically made by the patient describing a pain that starts in the central region of the abdomen and then spreads to the right iliac fossa. The pain of angina often radiates to the arm or jaw, and biliary colic occurs as pain in the upper abdomen that is referred to the back and is felt between the shoulder blades. Some skin conditions begin as single discrete lesions in one part of the body before spreading elsewhere, while others present in a more generalised way.

Incidence or frequency

If a symptom recurs, then in some circumstances the pattern of recurrence or relapse is characteristic. For example, classical migraine will rarely occur twice in the same week whereas another form of migraine, known as cluster headache, occurs every day at the same time of day for several weeks. The hay fever syndrome may often be difficult to distinguish from symptoms of the common cold except that it is notable for its appearance in particular months of the year.

Factors that relieve the condition

Just as some conditions are made worse by particular factors, there are some which can be characterised by factors which relieve them. The pain of peptic ulcer, for instance, is often relieved by small snacks (as opposed to large meals, which tend to aggravate it) and a migraine attack may be terminated by the patient vomiting.

Medicines are often useful to relieve and at the same time diagnose a condition. Thus, an anginal attack may be relieved by glyceryl trinitrate and reflux dyspepsia alleviated by a large dose of antacid, but not vice versa.

The intelligent use of a standard format such as the one we have suggested for asking questions will ensure that the most important areas are covered and that an acceptable standard of interrogation is used. The format we have used here will be applied as appropriate in the topics to be covered in this series, but as all practitioners will be aware, every question is not always applicable to every circumstance and the answer to one question often obviates the need for another. With practice, pharmacists will be able to use a standard line of questioning quickly and efficiently, knowing that as long as they have picked out the relevant questions for the symptom under consideration they will have acted in the best possible faith and with acceptable professional competency.

They will thus have been able to distinguish between minor illness and major disease. In practice, in many cases the cause of a symptom will be obvious while in others a precise diagnosis, at least prospectively, will be impossible and then the pharmacist will depend on the exclusion of serious pathology.

To complete the skill of diagnosis, even at this level, the pharmacist needs to rely on two further attributes. First, to have in mind a list of the serious diagnoses when considering the symptoms that are presented. Secondly, but no less importantly, to be alert to that unpleasant feeling which develops in a diagnostician's mind when no satisfactory explanation can be arrived at. This is a developed skill that many call experience. If any of the serious diagnoses cannot be reasonably excluded, the pharmacist should have no hesitation in directing the patient to more suitable assistance, e.g. referring to the doctor for a medical opinion.

It is important that pharmacists do not inadvertently raise fears in the minds of patients, especially when recommending referral to a doctor. Obviously it is both educative and consoling to be able to explain to a patient exactly why he or she should seek a medical opinion and there is no doubt that patients appreciate a sympathetic ear and a comprehensible explanation of both symptoms and their management. At the same time, when a pharmacist cannot eliminate the possibility of serious pathology from the patient's history it is essential that he/she delivers the message appropriately depending on the demeanour of the individual patient. Patients will often have selective hearing and overreact to emotive words such as 'cancer' or 'tumour', perhaps in such a way that they will then avoid seeing the doctor in case the diagnosis is confirmed. It is necessary to avoid the use of such words and to remember that statistically only a very small number of patients who seek help about their symptoms from a pharmacist will turn out to have serious disease and an even smaller proportion of symptoms will be due to malignancy. However, there will always be a few cases where there is a degree of uncertainty or where patients fall into a certain category in which it is good professional practice to advise them to take up the privilege available to them to see their doctor. The same process occurs daily in the doctor's consulting room where he/she will refer a patient for specialist opinion for similar reasons to either confirm or exclude specific diagnoses.

Format of this book

Each chapter in this book contains the main text, in which there is a description of commonly presenting signs and symptoms and their association with various diseases and conditions, together with advice to assist the pharmacist in interpreting them. Potential diagnoses and signals for referral are included as well as the principles of management with OTC medicines.

A summary of the most common conditions producing the described signs and symptoms is provided as well as a précis of the warning signals for referral.

Finally, a number of case histories are provided for illustration. These are based on real cases seen by the authors.

2

Headache

Headache is often no more than a physiological response to circumstance but it can lead to much anxiety, both for sufferers and for those who aim to unravel its cause. There are two major problems in attempting to discover the origin of a headache. Firstly, there are some potentially very serious diagnoses, which, although rare, may be in the minds of both parties, and secondly, it can be a notoriously difficult condition to explain. There are few definitive signs or tests available to either general practitioners or pharmacists that will confirm the diagnosis, yet headache is a common complaint which will bring many people to the pharmacy to purchase analgesics.

Fortunately, in most cases the headache will disappear spontaneously or respond to simple analgesics, proving, albeit retrospectively, to be no more than one of the transient self-limiting episodes to which most people are susceptible at some time or another. However, to distinguish the minority of cases in which serious pathology may be a possibility, it is helpful to understand the mechanisms by which headaches occur and to arrive at some guidelines to differentiate those types which may relate to an underlying problem from those which are of no lasting significance and can be treated symptomatically by the pharmacist.

Types

Tension headache

Tension headache is the most common cause of headache. It is sometimes referred to as psychogenic headache. It can be caused by various emotional stresses, such as tension, anx-iety or fatigue. Classically it is thought to result from muscle spasm in the neck and scalp (see Figure 2.1).

Vascular headache

Dilatation or constriction of blood vessels in and around the brain will produce pain. Vascular

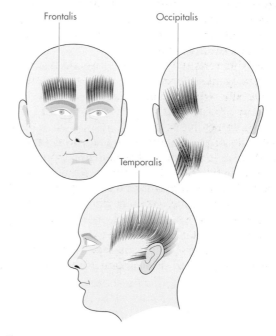

Figure 2.1 Location of the muscles of the scalp that are involved in muscular spasm in tension headache. When the muscles contract, there may be a tightness or band-like feeling around the head. Pain may be due in part to the tension in the muscles as well as a resulting constriction of capillaries within them, reducing their blood supply and causing a lack of oxygen.

headaches are the second most common cause of headache since this is the type associated with any febrile illness (which causes vaso-dilatation).

Hypertension rarely causes headache (although it is often believed to do so by patients with high blood pressure), except very rarely in severe or so-called malignant hypertension. The headache of migraine is due to dilatation of blood vessels within or around the skull. More serious cases of headache can be caused by rupture of a blood vessel, as in subarachnoid and subdural haemorrhages.

Traction headache

The brain itself has no sensory receptors within its fabric. A lesion within the substance of the brain will therefore not produce pain until it impinges upon adjacent structures, although if the lesion is severe enough to interfere with cerebral function, it may cause other symptoms such as vomiting, confusion, drowsiness or disturbances of balance or of intellectual function. Thus, even a lesion as severe as a stroke will not usually be accompanied by headache.

Traction headaches are caused by inflammation (e.g. meningitis), tumours or haematomas (haemorrhages). They are classified as traction headaches because the underlying pathology causes irritation and stretching of the meninges (the protective membranes enveloping the brain and spinal cord). These membranes are richly endowed with sensory pain receptors which, when stimulated, will cause headache.

Tumours and cerebral abscesses are examples of space-occupying lesions, which cause headaches by compressing normal brain tissue against the skull, resulting in a raised intracranial pressure. Head injury can cause a haematoma, leading to a raised intracranial pressure. Infection and inflammation of the membranes surrounding the brain and lining the skull (e.g. meningitis) will cause headache, as will inflammation of the brain tissue itself (e.g. encephalitis) when other structures are involved or the intracranial pressure rises.

Other causes

Headache can be caused by spasm or fatigue of the ciliary and periorbital muscles of the eye, as in eye strain, astigmatism and other refractive disorders. Glaucoma can cause headache. Pain may be referred from the jaw in dental pain and from the sinuses in sinusitis.

Muscle strain or pulled ligaments in the neck or upper back are a common cause of headache. Shingles affecting the scalp or eyes can cause pain in the face and head. Temporal arteritis is a rare but severe inflammation of the temporal artery and may occur in the elderly, producing pain and tenderness.

Assessing symptoms

Location of pain

Often headache cannot be described as pertaining to one part of the head, but if it is specific the following pointers are useful.

Frontal pain may indicate idiopathic headache (i.e. of no specific known cause), sinusitis or nasal congestion. Occipital pain (back of head) may suggest tension or anxiety, especially if the pain radiates over the top and sides of the head.

Tension headache is described as a tight band around the head, often spreading over the top of the head. It is usually bilateral and may be described by the patient as a generalised ache or pain, with no specific focus, felt all over the cranium.

Hemicranial (unilateral) headache, i.e. headache on one side of the head, is typical of migraine or sinusitis. It often spreads to both sides later. The pain of shingles (herpes zoster) usually starts as a severe localised pain felt in the skin on one side of the scalp, either a day or so before the rash appears or at the same time as the rash develops. Pain on one side of the face may indicate trigeminal neuralgia.

Pain from within the eye itself may be due to glaucoma or other serious eye diseases, but pain behind or around the eyes is often described in sinusitis, migraine or shingles.

Pain in the temple area (at the sides of the

head) may indicate temporal arteritis in patients over 50 years, especially if there is sensitivity to touch in this area of the scalp. This requires urgent referral to avoid more general inflammation of the arteries, which could lead to blindness if the blood supply to the optic nerve is compromised.

Radiation

As mentioned above, unilateral headaches such as migraine often subsequently spread to both sides of the head. It is important to remember to ask about the exact site and radiation of pain since transformation to a generalised headache might obscure the original pattern and location.

Duration and intensity

It is useful to ask the patient to assess the degree of pain suffered by asking the question 'How severe is the pain?' and then prompting the answer with 'Is it mild and annoying or is it severe and debilitating?' Another guide to severity is whether the patient is able to carry on with his/her daily routine.

It is helpful to know if the patient has suffered similar episodes before, since a new pain of some severity should be taken more seriously than recurrence of a headache which has been successfully dealt with in the past. Another useful question is 'Is this the worst pain you have ever had?' If the answer to this is yes, serious consideration should be given to referring the patient to the doctor.

If a headache has become progressively more severe over a period of days (or in the case of a child, a few hours) and is not responding to treatment, referral should be considered. A headache which is becoming less painful can reasonably be treated with simple analgesics, in the absence of any other significant factors.

A headache which has lasted only a few minutes can be regarded as trivial unless it has occurred suddenly and is described as devastating and the worst pain the patient has ever had. Such a headache might indicate bleeding from a ruptured blood vessel under the membrane covering the brain (subarachnoid haemorrhage) and is a medical emergency. Often the patient collapses and becomes unconscious under such circumstances. A migrainous headache can occur reasonably rapidly, but usually develops over a longer period than a subarachnoid haemorrhage, which may be described as being like a blow to the back of the head.

If a headache is of recent onset, but has gradually become worse over a few days, inquiry should be made about recent head trauma, since bleeding may occur slowly, giving progressive worsening of symptoms.

Migraine attacks classically last only a few hours but in some people they can persist for 72 hours.

The frequency as well as the duration of recurrent headaches should be noted and may reveal particular patterns. Classical and common migraine usually occur every few weeks and rarely more than once a week, whereas cluster headaches occur for one or two hours at the same time of day, every day, for several weeks.

Generally, a headache which does not disappear or improve over one to two weeks should be considered for referral with one or two exceptions, such as tension headache (which may occur every day for several weeks in some cases) and cluster headaches.

Nature of the symptom

A description of the pain can give valuable pointers to a possible cause of the headache. For example:

- **A sudden pain**, which feels like a blow to the head or an explosion in the head and which stops the patient in his/her tracks with no warning whatsoever suggests a haemorrhage (see above) and requires immediate referral, to a hospital if necessary, if the patient is in obvious distress.
- **Throbbing or pounding** indicates a vascular cause, e.g. fever or migraine.
- **Constant or nagging pain** is most probably due to a tension headache, but if it progressively worsens the possibility of something more serious should be borne in mind.

Table 2.1 Differentiation between migraine and tension headache

Migraine	Tension headache
Moderate to severe pain	Mild to moderate pain
Usually unilateral	Bilateral
Pulsating	Non-pulsating
Aggravated by normal activities, such that the patient has to stop	Not aggravated by normal actitivies

The pain of migraine is more severe than that of tension headache, but the most easily discriminating factors are the duration and the other associations such as nausea, vomiting or visual disturbances. Table 2.1 lists signs that differentiate tension headache from migraine.

If the patient complains of vague generalised pain, pressure on top or around the head or short stabbing pain, but does not have any other warning signs, a trial of OTC analgesics is reasonable.

Onset of pain/trigger factors

Establishing a pattern to the onset of headaches, especially recurrent episodes, can help not only in seeking a possible cause but also in removing trigger factors. When appropriate, inquiries based on the list shown in Table 2.2 will be helpful.

Table 2.2 Trigger factors for headache

Trigger factors or onset pattern	Possible underlying cause
Food, e.g. cheese, chocolate, caffeine, specific alcoholic drinks	Migraine
Exercise	Migraine, space-occupying lesion
Light	Migraine, meningitis
Hunger	Migraine
Neck movement	Tension, neck injury, meningitis, arthritis or fibrositis of the neck, vascular pathology
Cyclical pattern in females	Side effect of oral contraceptive, premenstrual tension, migraine, depression, tension
Present on awakening or wakes patient at night	Tension, neck muscle spasm, sinusitis, space-occupying lesion causing increased intracranial pressure
Bending down	Space-occupying lesion, sinusitis
Straining, coughing, sneezing	Space-occupying lesion
Sudden and severe with rapid onset	Subarachnoid haemorrhage
Travel	Tension, migraine
Drugs	Various, including oral contraceptives, indometacin, vasodilators (e.g. nitrates, calcium antagonists). Check BNF monographs for individual drugs
Ice cream, cold food	Usually no organic cause

Relieving factors

Avoidance of trigger factors can help in diagnosing the cause of a headache as well as relieving it. Migraine headaches are classically relieved by sleep or by vomiting.

Premenstrual syndrome, which may present with a headache and other symptoms (see below), classically improves or disappears when menstrual bleeding starts.

Accompanying symptoms

Inquiries about concurrent symptoms can help in differentiating between some types of headache.

Fever

A fever in adults with headache, especially with aching muscles (myalgia), aching joints and/or general malaise, is common in viral infections, sometimes accompanied by other symptoms of upper respiratory tract infection. Fever may also accompany the headache of sinusitis, along with nasal congestion or recent symptoms of the common cold and tenderness of the sinus areas to light finger pressure (see Figure 2.2). Fever may occasionally accompany the pain at the side of the head associated with temporal arteritis. In children, fever is one of the distinguishing factors in meningitis.

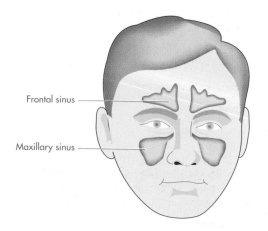

Frontal sinus

Maxillary sinus

Figure 2.2 Position of the frontal and maxillary sinuses.

Tender temples

Elderly patients can develop temporal arteritis, a condition in which either one or both of the temporal arteries are inflamed and may be seen as a red, congested vessel in the temple area, running vertically up the side of the head just in front of the ear. The patient will find that pressure applied to the skin over the artery is very painful. The patient with temporal arteritis may, rarely, have pain or an ache in the jaw, particularly after eating. This is due to obstruction of the blood supply from the cranial artery. If temporal arteritis is suspected, the patient requires same-day referral for a medical opinion.

Insomnia

If a headache is severe enough to interfere with sleep, the patient should seek a medical opinion, but more commonly patients will complain of early morning wakening or an inability to fall asleep on retiring, unrelated to the headache, and this may indicate depression and anxiety, respectively. Symptoms of tiredness, poor appetite and mood changes will point to the possibility of a tension headache.

Visual disturbances

Failing vision requires referral, but visual phenomena are a common feature of classical migraine or migraine with aura and constitute part of the aura which precedes the headache. Common migraine or migraine without aura describe migraine in which no such features are present. The visual symptoms of the aura of classical migraine can take the form of blurred vision, blind spots, flashing lights and zigzagging. They disappear within an hour and are followed by severe headache. Nausea frequently also occurs. Restriction of the visual field or the appearance of haloes around lights, especially in one eye only, suggest glaucoma or the optic neuritis of multiple sclerosis and same-day referral is required. Visual loss or double vision may occur in temporal arteritis. Any disturbance of vision, unless attributable to migraine, requires urgent referral of the patient.

It is noteworthy that only 10 to 20 per cent of

migraineurs have an aura of any description and therefore other causes of visual disturbance resembling the descriptions associated with migraine should be borne in mind and referral made if there is any uncertainty or the duration is longer than one hour. Such causes may be acute vascular or neurological deficits such as stroke, retinal occlusion or other intra-ocular pathology.

Neck stiffness

Neck stiffness in an adult with headache may be related to a neck strain or injury, but it could be a sign of a traction headache. Difficulty in being able to place the chin on the chest is a signal to refer urgently, particularly in children and young adults, since it raises the possibility of meningitis.

Nausea and vomiting

Nausea, with or without vomiting, is present in patients with migraine, glaucoma, space-occupying lesions and meningitis.

Nasal congestion and rhinitis

Nasal congestion accompanies the headache of sinusitis and is also seen in some patients with cluster headaches, together with rhinitis and facial flushing.

Central nervous system symptoms

Patients reporting signs and symptoms of involvement of the central nervous system require special consideration for referral. Symptoms may reflect general disturbances, such as loss of co-ordination and balance, drowsiness, irritability, personality changes and even fits. Sometimes the symptoms will reflect more localised lesions, such as slurred speech, muscle weakness in a limb and disturbances of the senses of smell and hearing. Such problems may accompany the headache of space-occupying lesions, such as tumours, and also subarachnoid haemorrhage and subdural haemorrhage (as in head injuries). Paraesthesia (pins and needles or numbness), usually in the arm, may occur as part of the aura of classical migraine, but this should disappear within a short time.

Any persistent unusual sensations require investigation as they may be a sign of a space-occupying lesion.

All of these conditions, with the exception of migraine, are rare, particularly in terms of presentation in the pharmacy. Nevertheless, they are potentially devastating diagnoses and must constantly be borne in mind.

Rash

In children or young adults with headache, the appearance of a rash anywhere on the body is a reason to refer immediately for a medical opinion to exclude meningitis. The meningococcal rash classically is purpuric, i.e. it is formed by haemorrhages from small blood vessels and leaves purple marks on the skin which do not blanch when pressed. However, in the early stages the presentation can be confusing.

Weight loss

Although the presentation in the pharmacy of weight loss (over a period of weeks or months) associated with headache will be unusual, it should always be regarded as a potentially serious sign, requiring referral. It may occur in cranial arteritis and systemic disease, as well as in patients with malignancy.

Other symptoms

Premenstrual syndrome in females, which may present as a monthly cyclical headache, can also occur in a variety of symptomatic presentations including irritability, anxiety and depression, bloating in the abdomen, breast tenderness, and swelling of the hands, ankles or feet.

Special considerations in children

As with all illnesses, it is difficult to obtain an exact history from a child and young children who feel ill may well describe their malaise as a headache without head pain being a feature at all.

Special attention should be paid to the possibility of a head injury, since young children receive more than their fair share of knocks.

Neck stiffness, which could be a sign of meningitis, should immediately alert the pharmacist to refer the patient but this symptom may be hard to elicit in young children. Meningitis is often notoriously difficult to diagnose, even by doctors, and it is essential that pharmacists should take the time to find out whether a child looks ill or behaves oddly, appears drowsy or irritable, or is vomiting or failing to feed.

The popular conception of meningitis is that of a sudden severe illness which is fatal if not immediately treated. This is true of the rare epidemic meningococcal forms. Rash is a danger signal but the symptoms do not all develop together and the 'warning' signs often occur relatively late on. The time from the first appearance of symptoms to a stage when the chance of survival is severely compromised can be as short as a few hours. However, viral meningitis often has a more insidious onset and could easily present, particularly in its early stages, in the pharmacy. Great caution is advised therefore in children with headaches. Where any doubts exist, same-day or more urgent referral (depending on the duration and severity) is mandatory.

Management

Removal of the underlying cause

Once serious pathology has been eliminated, consideration should be given to removing any possible predisposing factors or triggers.

Patients should be encouraged to persist for a week or so with any newly prescribed drugs suspected of causing the headache, since often an adjustment period is necessary, but this will depend on the severity of the headache. In most cases, alternative drugs will be available.

Non-drug methods

The treatment of chronic or repeated headaches, such as tension and migrainous types, lends itself to many types of non-drug therapy, such as massage, acupuncture, osteopathy and hypnotherapy.

OTC drugs

The response of individual patients to simple analgesics is variable because of both pharmacological and psychological factors.

Pain is a subjective, emotional symptom and treatment of chronic headache should be holistic rather than restricted to the symptom itself. The placebo effect is a valuable adjuvant to medication under such circumstances and a sympathetic ear and reassuring counsel will often help to alleviate the anxiety that is felt by some patients.

Soluble and effervescent formulations of analgesics, especially aspirin, will reduce the likelihood of gastrointestinal adverse effects. No clear correlation exists between the rapid attainment of so-called therapeutic blood levels and the onset of pain relief after ingestion of soluble tablet formulations, but the powerful placebo effect of effervescent tablets should not be ignored. They are also a rational choice in patients with migraine, since the reduced gut motility associated with this condition is thought to reduce and delay the absorption of drug from standard tablet formulations.

Citric acid, present in some effervescent formulations, can enhance aluminium absorption and produce toxicity in patients with chronic renal failure who are taking aluminium salts as a phosphate binder.

Paracetamol

Paracetamol, aspirin and ibuprofen have similar analgesic activity but paracetamol lacks the anti-inflammatory effects of the non-steroidal anti-inflammatory drugs. Paracetamol is a suitable analgesic to recommend when aspirin is contraindicated and generally enjoys a reputation as a safe drug in therapeutic doses. Interactions with warfarin have been reported, but at present there is not enough evidence to suggest avoiding its use in anticoagulated patients at normal doses.

Paediatric formulations of paracetamol are recommended for children.

Non-steroidal anti-inflammatory agents

Aspirin is one of the oldest OTC drugs. It provides adequate analgesia in most situations. It has anti-inflammatory properties and is therefore suitable for musculoskeletal causes of headache. Aspirin is contraindicated in children under 12 years of age because of its association with Reye's syndrome. It should not be recommended for patients with a history of peptic ulcer or dyspepsia. Five per cent of asthmatic patients are hypersensitive to aspirin and in its most severe form this allergy can manifest as a life-threatening asthmatic attack.

Aspirin has been widely used in pregnancy but it may cause problems in late pregnancy and paracetamol is regarded as the analgesic of choice.

Aspirin should not be recommended for patients who are taking anticoagulants nor for those already taking other non-steroidal anti-inflammatory drugs.

Ibuprofen is a relative newcomer to the OTC analgesic market in the UK, when compared with aspirin and paracetamol. Its actions and contraindications are similar to those of aspirin, but it may cause less gastric toxicity. Because of its more recent deregulation from the status of a prescription-only medicine, and because of its continuing popularity amongst doctors who continue to prescribe it, ibuprofen may be perceived as a more modern and powerful medicine than aspirin by the lay public. This useful placebo factor may be important when the pharmacist is deciding the most appropriate treatment for individual patients.

Combination products

Products that contain aspirin, paracetamol and codeine in various combinations can be seen as a second-line approach for use when single component products fail to alleviate symptoms.

Although the evidence for increased clinical analgesia with these drug combinations is minimal, particularly with codeine at a dose of 8 mg, there is a tendency for both the public and health professionals alike to consider them as more powerful than single agents. This is not totally irrational, and no doubt their use is a successful ploy in the management of many patients.

Codeine can cause constipation and continued dosing should be avoided where this might be problematic, such as in the elderly.

Caffeine is often present in analgesic combinations and is claimed to potentiate the activity and the absorption of analgesics. The data to support the clinical significance of these actions are equivocal and, theoretically, caffeine can be harmful since it may stimulate secretion of gastric acid (enhancing the irritant effect of aspirin) and cause central excitation (counteracting the desire to obtain relief of headache by rest or sleep in some patients, particularly in migraine).

Feverfew

Feverfew is a herbal remedy which has had variable success in the prophylaxis of migraine. It can be regarded at best to be of modest benefit, but some patients appear to do well on it. It has definite pharmacological activity on prostaglandin synthesis and platelet aggregation but it is unclear whether these mechanisms are significant in migraine. Feverfew is contraindicated in pregnancy because of its stimulant effect on uterine muscle.

Special considerations

Migraine

Gastric motility is reduced during a migraine attack and it is thought that this causes impaired absorption of oral analgesics. It is essential therefore that analgesics be taken at the first sign of an attack and preferably in the form of a soluble or effervescent product to expedite absorption. This is an important point to stress to patients in order to maximise the effect of treatment.

Some proprietary products that are recommended specifically for migraine contain antihistamines, such as cyclizine and buclizine, which are included presumably for their antiemetic effect. Additionally, some antihistamines do have analgesic activity and their inclusion in migraine products may be logical in this respect.

Table 2.3   Interactions between OTC analgesics and prescribed drugs

OTC analgesic	Interacting drug	Consequence
Aspirin	Anticoagulants, e.g. warfarin	Extended clotting time, potential haemorrhages
Aspirin Paracetamol Codeine	Prescribed drugs and combination products containing the same individual components, e.g. co-proxamol, co-codamol	Additive toxicity
Aspirin	Methotrexate	Renal excretion of methotrexate reduced
Ibuprofen	Lithium	Renal excretion of lithium reduced

Dental pain

Dental pain can be partially or temporarily alleviated by simple analgesics, although persistent pain will not be affected and requires referral to a dentist (see Chapter 16). Following dental surgery, however, aspirin should be avoided because of its antiplatelet activity, which may prolong bleeding.

Drug interactions

Major drug interactions between OTC analgesics and prescribed drugs are highlighted in Table 2.3.

SUMMARY OF CONDITIONS PRODUCING HEADACHE

Dental pain
Dental pain, especially pain emanating from the jaw, can radiate to the head.

Glaucoma
An increase in intraocular pressure can cause headache, pain from within the eye, haloes around lights, defective vision, red eye, dilated pupils and vomiting – **refer**.

Haemorrhage
Subdural haemorrhage may follow a head injury. Symptoms may appear immediately, or at any time for several weeks. They worsen progressively and as well as headache there may be drowsiness and sometimes numbness on one side of the body – **refer**.

Subarachnoid haemorrhage is not usually associated with head injury. It occurs suddenly like a devastating blow to the occipital area, often causing collapse. The patient will show obvious signs of confusion and will be severely ill – **refer**.

(continued overleaf)

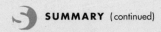 **SUMMARY** (continued)

Meningitis
Most common in children but also occurs in teenagers and young adults. Symptoms include headache, fever, photophobia, nausea or vomiting, irritability or drowsiness, confusion and neck stiffness. Skin rash (often appears late) presents as bruise-like spots which do not blanch on pressure from fingers. The patient may deteriorate over a few hours and become very ill – **refer**.

Migraine
Classical migraine with aura
This is characterised by an aura which lasts for up to one hour preceding the headache. The aura consists of mainly visual disturbances such as blurred vision, blind spots or flashing and zigzag lights. Sometimes there is numbness or paraesthesia, usually in an arm. After the aura, the headache develops, initially on one side but it may spread quickly to become bilateral. It lasts for several hours and is usually accompanied by nausea and sometimes photophobia. The attack often ends with the patient vomiting. A period of resolution follows, during which the patient may feel tired and lethargic, before recovery is complete. Migraine attacks usually recur at intervals of more than one or two weeks. Now often known as migraine with aura.

Common migraine, or migraine without aura
Ninety per cent of migraineurs suffer from common migraine, which resembles the classical type except that there is no aura.

Cluster headaches
These are so-called because they occur in clusters, lasting an hour or two, at the same time of day or night and recur every day for several weeks. The pain is usually around one eye and there is lacrimation and/or a congested or runny nose.
   Migraine can often be alleviated by simple analgesics. If unsuccessful, medical referral should be made to consider use of the many drug treatments which are available on prescription only.

for diagnos
of pontis

Premenstrual syndrome (premenstrual tension)
A syndrome which presents in females in a variety of forms, often with headache. It is characterised by its regular cyclical appearance, usually commencing seven to ten days before menstruation and disappearing or at least improving when bleeding occurs. Other common symptoms include irritability, anxiety and depression, loss of concentration, abdominal bloating, breast tenderness, swelling of the hands, feet or ankles, and weight gain.

Refractive errors
Patients requiring correction of vision or suffering from eye strain may suffer from headaches.

Shingles (herpes zoster infection)
Infection of nerve tracts in the face or scalp with the herpes zoster virus causes a rash accompanied by shooting pain. Severe pain, often over an eye or one half of the scalp or face, occurs and may persist for several weeks after the rash has healed (post-herpetic neuralgia) – **refer**.

Sinusitis
Headache may be unilateral or bilateral, and is often accompanied by a head cold or nasal congestion.

→

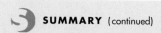 **SUMMARY** (continued)

There may be a green, purulent nasal discharge. The skin over the sinuses (around the orbit of the eye) is sensitive to pressure applied by the fingers.

Space-occupying lesion (e.g. brain abscess, tumour)
Headache is caused by a raised intracranial pressure due to the expanding intracerebral mass. The pain may at first respond to simple analgesics, but becomes progressively more severe over several weeks. It is accompanied by other central nervous system disturbances (depending on the part of the brain involved) such as mood change, drowsiness, slurred speech, loss of balance or co-ordination, vomiting, limb weakness or strange sensations of taste or smell. The headache is classically worse on awakening and is exacerbated by the raised intracranial pressure produced by coughing, sneezing, straining, bending over, etc. – **refer**.

Temporal arteritis
A disease of the elderly, temporal arteritis is an inflammation of the temporal artery, which traverses the side of the head just in front of the ear. The condition is part of a more extensive cranial arteritis which is an inflammatory process affecting various blood vessels supplying the brain. It is usually seen in patients who suffer from polymyalgia rheumatica, a collagen vascular disease which presents with morning joint stiffness, pain and weakness, affecting primarily the neck, shoulders, back and thighs. The head pain is usually unilateral and severe and the temporal artery may be red, prominent and exquisitely tender to the touch. Sometimes there may be jaw pain after eating because of reduced circulation to the jaw muscles. This disease requires same-day referral since it can lead to blindness if the ophthalmic arteries become affected. The diagnosis can only be confirmed by biopsy of the artery – **refer.**

Tension
Tension headache is the most common type of headache in people aged under 50 years. Causative factors, such as stress, are sometimes easily elicited, but they are not always obvious. Classically, the headache is described as a tight band around the head, spreading over the top of the scalp, but its distribution can also be more vague and generalised or located at the back of the head or around the eyes. It can persist for several weeks and is notoriously difficult to treat with simple analgesics. It usually resolves spontaneously. Tricyclic antidepressants have been reported to be helpful in some cases.

Trauma
Headache following a head injury may exist as a localised pain in the first few hours but continues as a generalised headache. It may be caused by a subdural haemorrhage (see above), concussion or fracture, and may result in disturbances such as drowsiness, dizziness, slurred speech, nausea and vomiting. The pupils may be of unequal size and may fail to react to light – **refer**.

Trigeminal neuralgia
A rare presentation, trigeminal neuralgia occurs chiefly from middle age onwards. It often takes the form of a sharp, excruciating pain on one side of the face, lasting a few seconds, and is triggered by touching a sensitive area on the face. Sometimes the pain is accompanied by involuntary movements in the distribution of the affected nerve. It is not in itself a danger to life, but it requires treatment with specific drugs such as carbamazepine – **refer**.

WHEN TO REFER
Headache

Onset/severity
- Sudden, explosive, patient 'stopped in tracks' → Immediate referral
- Occurring some time after a head injury → Immediate referral
- Obvious severity: disabling, patient cannot move, interferes with daily routine (and patient not experienced this before), patient appears ill   Same day/immediate*

Frequency and duration
- Unremitting
- Progressively worsening over weeks
- Short duration but worsening over days

Accompanying symptoms   → Pins x needles
- Nausea/vomiting   Same day/immediate*
- Neurological signs, e.g. paraesthesia, mood change, drowsiness, slurred speech, loss of balance, irritability and poor co-ordination   Same day/immediate*
- Visual disturbance (if migraine has been excluded)   Same day/immediate*
- Pupils unequal in size or not responding to light   Same day/immediate*
- Loss of consciousness   Same day/immediate*
- Jaw pain   Same day
- Tenderness over temples   Same day
- Neck stiffness   Immediate
- Rash
  - on scalp in adult   Same day
  - on skin in child or young adult   Immediate

Pattern
- Worse on awakening

Location of pain
- Temporal area   Same day/immediate*
- Focussed above or lateral to eye   Same day/immediate*

*Urgency of referral is a matter of judgement, depending on the signs and symptoms

CASE STUDIES

Case 1

A slim woman presents to the pharmacist wanting something for her headache. She appears to be in her early 30s, is wearing jeans and a sweater, and has two young children with her, who are not well behaved around the shop.

The headache has been present intermittently for several weeks, and is dull, central or sometimes occipital, feeling like a tight band around her head. It is unrelated to food, exercise or posture, although a cigarette often eases it. It interrupts her at night occasionally, being especially present in the evenings, making it difficult for her to get to sleep. She has consulted a doctor, and is living at present with her parents after the breakdown of her marriage.

A combination of codeine and paracetamol is recommended, and on her return about two weeks later to seek advice about one of her children she reports success with the medication, particularly at night. A better night's sleep has helped her to unwind and consider her future more objectively.

Both she and the pharmacist agree that the headache could be attributed to stress.

Case 2

A retired man seeks the advice of his pharmacist. Since leaving the civil service some eight years ago he has enjoyed a peaceful retirement, although recently he has been troubled by headaches. They are vague, nowhere in particular, but are progressively worse with time. He is reluctant to consult his doctor, believing, or at least hoping, there is nothing serious amiss.

On more detailed and systemic questioning it emerges that his appetite is poor, he has lost probably a stone in weight and he has felt generally unwell for more than six months. There are few specific symptoms, but he has become increasingly breathless in the last four to six weeks.

The pharmacist is unsure of the diagnosis, but spends some time encouraging the patient to have further investigations. This he apparently does, for three weeks later his wife brings in a prescription for the newly diagnosed renal failure. Whilst she is anxious as to the prognosis, she remains grateful to the pharmacist for directing her husband to much needed help.

Case 3

A woman in her mid 40s tells her pharmacist she has tension headaches. They are usually stress induced, and are often premenstrual. They are almost always left sided, and although insidious in onset are often accompanied by nausea. She has tried paracetamol, but has found that the best relief is to lie quietly in a darkened room. The light hurts her eyes, and she can often sleep off the headache, if the family let her. The pharmacist feels this is very likely to be migraine. She is taking no medication, has had a recent eye test and has not seen her doctor for two years. She persuades the pharmacist to recommend analgesia and the pharmacist in turn asks her to return to report the outcome.

About a month later she returns. She has taken the medicine as advised, especially at the start of the headache, but with little and only temporary effect. She would like something stronger, but is persuaded to see her doctor. The doctor finally wins her confidence by explaining how the treatment of migraine has improved with specific prescription therapies.

3

Cough

Cough is a reflex which is stimulated by irritation of the respiratory mucosa in the lungs, the trachea or the pharynx. It is often a reaction to infection or contamination of the respiratory tract and is a protective mechanism to clear the airways of contaminants.

It may be desirable sometimes to encourage a cough and sometimes to suppress it.

Types

Coughs may be broadly described as either productive, i.e. producing sputum, or non-productive (dry), with no sputum.

Assessing symptoms

Productive or non-productive

A non-productive cough may be described as dry, tickly or irritating. It produces no sputum and generally the pharmacist can be reassured that the cause is unlikely to be bacterial infection, although this must be considered along with other symptoms. In some circumstances patients will deny bringing up any sputum, although they will say that they can feel phlegm on their chest. In such cases, the cough is best regarded as productive rather than non-productive.

Non-productive coughs are irritating, not only to the patient, but also to those who live or work with him or her. They occur as a typical response to damage of the epithelium of the upper respi-ratory tract caused by viral infection, smoking (active and passive), a dry atmosphere, air pollution (especially in the workplace) or a change in temperature. They may also be a feature of some serious conditions such as asthma or lung cancer, or an adverse reaction to drugs, e.g. ACE inhibitors.

In a patient with a productive cough, the appearance of the sputum can be helpful in eliciting the severity of any underlying cause.

Sputum

Clear or white sputum can be considered generally as being of little significance, unless produced in copious amounts.

Thick yellow, green or brown sputum or foul-smelling sputum suggests a lower respiratory (i.e. lung) infection, such as bronchitis. Clear, straw-coloured sputum may be seen in disorders of allergic origin, such as some forms of asthma, the yellow tinge being caused by the presence of large quantities of eosinophil cells from the blood as part of the allergic response.

Blood in the sputum (haemoptysis) may be seen as either copious fresh blood, spots or streaks and sometimes it may discolour the sputum brown. It should be regarded with suspicion and referral suggested for further investigation since it may be a sign of pulmonary embolism, tuberculosis, bronchitis or lung cancer. Check that the blood does appear to be coming from the lung and not from the mouth, throat or nose (caused by trauma, such as nose blowing).

Pink and frothy sputum is sometimes seen in heart failure, where there is congestion of blood in the lungs and some leakage of plasma into the air spaces.

Patients with pneumonia typically produce rust-coloured sputum at first, which may progress to being blood stained.

Duration and frequency

Coughs are usually self-limiting. Any patient with a cough which has lasted more than two weeks without improvement requires referral. Recurrent coughs may indicate a serious problem requiring referral. For instance, patients with chronic bronchitis suffer persistent coughs for more than three months in the year and patients with bronchiectasis have recurrent chest infections and require antibiotics. Cigarette smokers often have a recurrent cough, which may be due to chronic bronchitis, and they should be examined by their doctor to exclude infection or lung damage.

Long-standing or recurrent cough, especially in patients over 40 years of age, may be a sign of more sinister disease such as lung cancer.

Onset

The onset of a cough may be sudden, acute and devastating, causing collapse or serious illness, as is the case in pneumonia. More often, however, the onset is slower and less dramatic. If it occurs at night and is accompanied by catarrh it may be caused by a postnasal drip (see below). The cough of bronchitis or bronchiectasis is worse on awakening.

Most coughs are worse at night but special care should be taken to identify a dry night-time cough in children, which could possibly be due to asthma, and night-time cough and breathlessness in adults, which indicate possible pulmonary congestion, as seen in heart failure.

Accompanying symptoms

Nasal congestion, sore throat, fever, myalgia

Cough is commonly associated with or preceded by symptoms of the common cold or influenza-like illnesses. In such cases it is invariably nothing more than a simple viral infection, which may be treated symptomatically with OTC drugs.

Shortness of breath, difficulty in breathing (dyspnoea)

These symptoms should alert the pharmacist to refer the patient to the doctor. Such symptoms may be progressive over a number of months or years, indicating chronic bronchitis, emphysema, heart failure or other serious disease, or they may be recurrent, as in asthma, when the characteristic wheeze may be heard. A sudden onset of breathlessness occurs in pneumothorax, pulmonary embolism and pleurisy.

Chest pain

The lung tissue itself has no sensory pain fibres. Pain felt in the chest caused by respiratory disease can arise from the pleura, trachea, bronchi or the vascular supply. Such pain always requires immediate referral. Pain felt on deep inspiration or coughing may be caused by pleurisy or pulmonary embolism. Intercostal muscle strain following a coughing bout also produces these symptoms and can be difficult to distinguish from pleuritic pain.

Fever

Fever and sweating in a patient with cough suggests infection.

Weight loss

A dramatic loss of weight suggests the possibility of serious disease such as tuberculosis or lung cancer.

Painful calf

Pain in the calf muscles, possibly associated with swelling in the calf or ankle, may be caused by a deep vein thrombosis; there may also be signs of skin inflammation. The thrombus may break up and be transported by the circulation to the pulmonary artery where it will lodge as a pulmonary embolus, causing a pulmonary infarct. Chest pain is the predominant feature, along with shortness of breath, but a cough may also be present.

Special considerations: age

In patients over 40 years of age, serious lung disease should be considered, especially if cough has been present for many years. The possibility of chronic bronchitis and some of the consequences of repeated infection and damage to the lung, such as bronchiectasis and emphysema, should alert the pharmacist to refer the patient, especially when other symptoms suggest a serious diagnosis. In patients of this age, especially if they are smokers, the possibility of lung cancer should always be considered.

Children between the ages of about four and eight years may suffer from the catarrhal child syndrome. Such patients experience repeated colds and catarrh, often accompanied by earache. At night, catarrh may run down the back of the throat, irritating the pharyngeal mucosa (postnasal drip) to produce a cough. Treatment is symptomatic. The child and its parents should be reassured that antibiotics will be of no use and that the episode will be self-limiting, although recurrence is likely until the child grows out of the condition at about eight years of age. Obviously, any doubts about a child who appears ill or who has had a cough for a number of days should prompt a referral to the doctor.

Young children between the ages of six months and two years who wake in the middle of the night with a barking or croaking cough may be suffering from croup. Symptoms usually abate the next morning but may recur the following night. If breathing is noisy (stridor) or there is a wheeze, urgent referral is required. Croup can cause narrowing of the airway because of oedema and so should be taken seriously. The condition can be difficult to differentiate from epiglottitis, in which the child appears ill, has difficulty in breathing and stridor, and attempts to sit or lean forward to breathe. Epiglottitis is a rare condition, but is potentially very serious. On inspecting the throat, a bright pink lump may sometimes be seen at the back, behind the tongue. If suspected, epiglottitis requires an emergency referral to hospital.

Drug-induced cough or breathlessness

A drug history can sometimes elicit the cause of a cough. For example, ACE inhibitors cause a dry cough in some patients and beta-blockers may precipitate heart failure, characterised by breathlessness, with or without a cough.

Management

There is a plethora of proprietary OTC cough medicines and making a suitable choice can present some difficulty to both the pharmacist and potential consumer. Doubts have been cast on the pharmacological activity of cough medicines and many doctors would say that it makes little difference to the course of a cough whether such a medicine is taken or not.

Like any other trivial symptom, a cough with no serious underlying cause will be self-limiting and will disappear spontaneously within a few days. However, public expectations are high and if someone comes into the pharmacy complaining of a cough, then there is a role for a 'cough bottle', even if it is little more than a placebo.

The confusion about cough medicines and the negative opinion among medical authorities about their efficacy is primarily related to the lack of clinical trials carried out to establish any useful clinical effects. Nevertheless, bearing in mind that many cough preparations do contain drugs with recognised pharmacological activity, it is pertinent to consider some logical rationale which can be applied when choosing a product to give symptomatic relief.

The cough mechanism

The cough reflex is a protective mechanism and in many cases interference with it may delay its disappearance or exacerbate the underlying disturbance which caused it.

The reflex has three nervous components: (a) receptors in the mucosa of the respiratory tract are sensitive to chemical or mechanical stimulation and activate the discharge of afferent impulses along cholinergic (vagus) nerve fibres to (b) the cough centre in the brain stem; (c) efferent impulses from the cough centre are then transmitted along cholinergic nerves to cause contraction of the diaphragm, abdominal and intercostal muscles, resulting in a rapid expulsion of air from the lungs, taking with it mucus and irritating particles on the surface of the respiratory mucosa.

OTC drugs

The active ingredients of cough medicines can be broadly classified into three groups.

Cough suppressants

Cough suppressants can usefully provide symptomatic relief of a dry, irritating or tickly cough which produces little or no sputum. A dry, tickly cough may be caused by an irritable mucous membrane in the upper respiratory tract resulting from oedema of the mucosa in the pharynx following a sore throat, or from mucus dripping from the postnasal space, which irritates the pharynx and trachea (postnasal drip).

Non-productive cough is common in tracheitis, in viral infections such as the common cold and in chronic bronchitis, at times where little sputum is produced. It can be distressing and exhausting, preventing sleep at night and irritating other people by day. Cough suppressants may act at different sites in the cough pathway.

Centrally acting cough suppressants Centrally acting cough suppressants act on the cough centre in the brain and reduce the discharge of impulses down the efferent nerves to the muscles which produce coughing. Examples are codeine, pholcodine and dextromethorphan. All are capable of causing sedation and long courses will give rise to constipation and may produce dependence. Thus, short courses only should be recommended.

Pholcodine and dextromethorphan reputedly have fewer adverse effects and less abuse potential than codeine. For these reasons, they are to be preferred and codeine should only be recommended in exceptional circumstances.

Antihistamines Antihistamines owe their antitussive properties more to their intrinsic anticholinergic activity than to any effect on histamine. They reduce the cholinergic transmission of impulses in the nervous pathway of the cough reflex and thus act as a cough sedative or suppressant. Examples of antihistamines which are commonly present in cough medicines include diphenhydramine, promethazine and triprolidine.

Antihistamines are not suitable for a productive cough. Arguments that they are unsuitable for patients with asthma because they may increase the viscosity of bronchial secretions are controversial and may not be of clinical significance. They are particularly helpful when a cough and a head cold coexist, since the antihistimine will also dry the nasal secretions that may cause a postnasal drip and initiate cough.

Antihistamines used in cough medicines can cause sedation and because of their anticholinergic properties they should be avoided by patients with narrow-angle glaucoma or enlarged prostate glands.

Demulcents Demulcents, such as honey, glycerin and syrup, are said to act by coating the pharyngeal mucosa, which may be inflamed, and offer some protection from irritants such as smoke or dust particles. Their efficacy probably relates largely to a soothing placebo effect, but the demulcent effect on the mucosa may be a real one and may also serve to hydrate the delicate mucosal tissues. Where postnasal drip occurs, demulcents may reduce irritation of the pharyngeal mucosa.

Expectorants

Expectorants increase bronchial secretions and thus reduce the tenacity of mucus, which can then be coughed up. They have a traditional place in cough therapy but their efficacy is controversial owing to a lack of strong supportive, objective data, although there is considerable subjective support for their use.

Plugs of mucus and debris in the small airways can cause breathing difficulties and act as sites of infection and patients who attempt to remove sputum which they can 'feel' in their chests may become exhausted by coughing if the mucus is so viscous that it adheres to the mucosal lining of the lungs. There are therefore good reasons for facilitating expectoration.

Hydration of the airways will ensure adequate production of non-viscous mucus from the glands lining the lungs. This can be simply and effectively achieved by drinking plenty of fluid, so that the tissues remain hydrated, as well as by humidifying the inspired air by using steam inhalations.

The addition of substances such as menthol or compound tincture of benzoin (Friar's balsam) to the hot water which provides the steam is probably of no extra value except for a psychological effect.

Expectorant agents used in cough medicines are thought to act by irritating the gastric mucosa, which produces a reflex stimulation of the bronchial tree. The latter responds by secreting more mucus.

Ammonium salts Various ammonium salts have been used over the years but the chloride is the most commonly used nowadays.

Guaifenesin This agent is present in many proprietary cough medicines although the dosage varies considerably. It would be logical to recommend doses of 100 to 200 mg for maximum effect.

Ipecacuanha Ipecacuanha stimulates the gastric mucosa at sub-emetic doses and enhances bronchial secretion.

Other expectorants Citric acid and sodium citrate have expectorant properties but these are probably weak in the doses used. Squill is an old established medicine which may be found in some proprietary cough remedies. Creosote, menthol and eucalyptol are oils which are thought to stimulate expectoration.

Bronchodilators

Sympathomimetic agents such as phenylpropanolamine, ephedrine and pseudoephedrine are used to relax bronchial smooth muscle. They are also useful as nasal decongestants and can therefore be recommended when a cough and nasal congestion occur together. Because of their vasoconstrictor effect, sympathomimetic agents should not be used by hypertensive patients, those with heart disease or those taking beta-blocking drugs or MAO inhibitors.

Theophylline is available in a few cough remedies in the UK. Its exact mode of action is unclear but it is an effective bronchodilator. The effective and safe dosage is very variable between patients and requires individualisation.

The small amounts of theophylline present in proprietary formulations are most likely subtherapeutic for most adults in the doses recommended, but they do at least appear to be safe. However, inquiry should always be made as to whether patients have been prescribed theophylline by their doctor; if this is the case, they should not take any more in OTC medicines since the additive effect of further doses could be toxic.

Combination cough mixtures

The majority of cough remedies contain mixtures of agents, often from different pharmacological classes. This in itself is perfectly acceptable, provided that individual constituents do not interact in an adverse manner. Unfortunately, this is has not been the case with some OTC cough medicines in the past and some appeared totally illogical from a pharmacological point of view. Fortunately, the number of such irrational combinations has declined in recent years. It might be argued that since there is little clinical evidence to support the efficacy of the individual drugs used, then the selection of one mixture in preference to another will be of no consequence. If, however, we have any faith in the preparations on the pharmacy shelves, it is imperative that the pharmacist's product recommendation is based on rational reasoning, from a pharmacological point of view. For example, combinations of expectorants and cough suppressants, or expectorants and antihistamines are irrational. If a cough is productive and requires an expectorant, then it should not be suppressed at the same time. Similarly, antihistamine drugs will reduce bronchial secretions by an anticholinergic mechanism and this is pharmacologically antagonistic to the effect of an expectorant. Some combinations are entirely logical. For example, a mixture of a bronchodilator and an expectorant, or a bronchodilator and a cough suppressant/antihistamine do not present any obvious pharmacological antagonism (see Tables 3.1 and 3.2).

Special considerations

Children and pregnant women

Because of the self-limiting nature of the majority of coughs and the controversial efficacy of cough medicines, it is advisable to recommend only demulcent syrups to young children and pregnant women. In some instances, where a child has an irritating cough, an antihistamine, such as promethazine syrup (Phenergan), will serve the double purpose of cough suppressant and sedative, to allow the patient (and the parents) to have a good night's sleep.

Patients with diabetes

Except in patients with poor control of their diabetes, short courses of cough medicines containing sugar will have no clinically significant effect

Table 3.1   Examples of pharmacologically rational mixtures

Suppressant	Bronchodilator/decongestant	Antihistamine
Dextromethorphan	Ephedrine	
Dextromethorphan	Pseudoephedrine	Diphenhydramine
Dextromethorphan	Pseudoephedrine	Triprolidine
Codeine	Pseudoephedrine	Brompheniramine
Pholcodine	Ephedrine	Chlorpheniramine (chlorphenamine)

Table 3.2   Examples of pharmacologically irrational mixtures

Expectorant	Suppressant	Antihistamine
Ammonium chloride		Diphenhydramine
Ammonium chloride	Dextromethorphan	Diphenhydramine
Ammonium chloride	Morphine	
Guaifenesin		Brompheniramine
Guaifenesin	Codeine	
Guaifenesin	Dextromethorphan	
Guaifenesin		Triprolidine

Table 3.3   Interactions between OTC cough medicines and prescribed drugs

OTC product	Interacting drug	Consequence
Antihistamines	Anxiolytics Hypnotics Sedatives Alcohol	Enhancement of sedative and CNS depressant effects
Antihistamines (because of intrinsic anticholinergic properties)	Phenothiazines Tricyclic antidepressants	Enhanced anticholinergic effects, e.g. blurred vision, dry mouth
Sympathomimetics	Antihypertensive therapy	Reduced antihypertensive effect
	MAOIs	Hypertensive crisis
	Tricyclic antidepressants	Hypertension possible with phenylephrine (less likely with phenylpropanolamine and ephedrine)
Theophylline	Cimetidine Erythromycin Quinolone antibacterial agents	Increased blood levels and risk of theophylline toxicity

in either insulin-dependent or non-insulin-dependent diabetes. If in any doubt, however, there are a few sugar-free cough medicines which can be recommended. Pharmacists should remember that patients with insulin-dependent diabetes may require more insulin when they have a bacterial or viral infection, even if they have lost their appetite. This is because excess adrenaline and other hormones with an anti-insulin effect are secreted in response to the stress of the infection.

Drug interactions

Major drug interactions between the ingredients of OTC cough medicines and prescribed medicines are shown in Table 3.3.

SUMMARY OF CONDITIONS PRODUCING COUGH

Asthma

Asthma is characterised by wheezing caused by bronchoconstriction, hypersecretion of mucus and inflammation of the bronchi. There is difficulty in breathing, particularly on expiration, so that patients feel that they cannot remove all the air from the lungs.

Asthma may be caused by allergens (extrinsic asthma) or may show no relation to obvious allergens (intrinsic asthma). It may be triggered by respiratory infection, air pollution or drugs such as beta-blockers. Acute attacks are sudden in onset, common during the night and, in children, they may present as a persistent dry cough. Attacks are usually relieved within a couple of hours. The sputum may be straw coloured because of the presence of eosinophils – **refer**.

(continued overleaf)

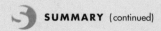 **SUMMARY** (continued)

Bronchiectasis

Repeated infections of the lung, such as occur in chronic bronchitis, will eventually lead to irreparable tissue damage. If such damage affects the terminal bronchioles, they become dilated and distorted in shape and their normal mucosal lining is replaced by scar tissue. This scar tissue cannot transport oxygen from the air in the lung to the blood, leading to increased respiratory distress. Cough is persistent and the sputum is purulent, more plentiful in the morning and occasionally blood stained. Inflammation and mucus plugs in the small bronchioles predispose to episodes of pneumonia – **refer**.

Bronchitis

Acute bronchitis is an infection of the bronchi which is usually bacterial and should be treated with antibiotics. The problem is that many coughs are labelled as bronchitis, and treated as such, when in fact they are bronchiolitis (irritant inflammation of the trachea and bronchi) or simply coughs associated with upper respiratory infections. Acute bronchitis may occur secondarily to upper respiratory viral infections, such as the common cold and influenza, or as an exacerbation of chronic bronchitis. Cough and chest soreness are present and the sputum is purulent. Patients will have chest tightness, wheeziness or difficulty in breathing. Often fever is present and occasionally the sputum may be blood stained – **refer**.

Chronic bronchitis results from repeated trauma to the lower respiratory tract and is often the end result of recurrent attacks of acute bronchitis. As well as infection, it may be caused by irritants such as tobacco smoke, atmospheric pollution, dust and irritants in the working environment. Social factors, such as overcrowding in the home, dampness or poor air conditioning, may predispose to chronic bronchitis. It is characteristically seen in middle age and beyond, and is more common in men than women. The patient will have had acute attacks of bronchitis which have increased in length and severity over the years. Gradually the cough fails to disappear between acute attacks and becomes persistent, referred to often by the patient as a smoker's cough. Damage to the lungs occurs and the patient has permanent symptoms, such as breathing difficulties, wheeze and shortness of breath. The disease may progress and cause death or it may become clinically static – **refer**.

Cancer of the lung

Cough, weight loss and dyspnoea are common symptoms of lung cancer. It is more common in men than women, usually appears between the ages of 50 and 70 years and is seen more often in cigarette smokers. Cough may have been present for some time in smokers, but any change in its character is a sign to refer. Blood in the sputum is commonly seen – **refer**.

Croup

The term 'croup' is used loosely by both medical and non-medical people to encompass a variety of symptoms associated with an irritant cough in children. Properly used, the term describes an infection (usually viral) of the larynx and trachea which leads to oedema and narrowing of the airway. There is a severe and violent cough, which is often paroxysmal (occurring in bouts). The child often has difficulty in breathing between bouts and stridor (noisy inspiration) is often present. The condition requires urgent medical appraisal – **refer**.

Emphysema

Recurrent trauma of infection and inflammation, as occurs in chronic bronchitis, can cause hyperinflation of the alveoli, leaving balloon-like processes called bullae, which are not able to transfer oxygen

→

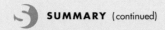 **SUMMARY** (continued)

efficiently across the lung wall. The bullae disintegrate progressively. Dyspnoea occurs, first on exertion and ultimately at rest, with other symptoms such as wheezing and a productive cough. If the bullae are ruptured at the surface of the lung into the pleural space, a pneumothorax may ensue – **refer**.

Pneumonia
Pneumonia is usually caused by bacterial infection, producing inflammatory changes (consolidation) in the lung tissue. It has a sudden onset, with a high temperature and cough, and the patient rapidly becomes ill. Chest pain will develop because of inflammation spreading to the pleural membranes which line the lung and chest wall. This pain, characteristic of pleuritic pain, is worse on deep inspiration and on coughing. The cough is initially unproductive but, as the disease progresses, purulent, rust-coloured and, later, blood-stained sputum is produced. Viral pneumonia, which often follows an upper respiratory infection, is more insidious in both onset and course; it should be thought of when a cough or other respiratory symptoms persist – **refer**.

Pneumothorax
The lung is normally held against the thoracic wall by a negative pressure in the pleural space that 'sucks' it out to assume the shape of the thoracic cavity. If the pleural envelope is ruptured, air enters into the pleural cavity, neutralising the negative pressure and as a result the lung collapses. This is a pneumothorax. It occurs without warning and for no apparent reason, particularly in healthy young men, as well as in bronchitis or emphysema. It gives rise to a severe, unilateral chest pain which may be either constant or pleuritic in nature and there may be some dyspnoea. The pain may be felt over the shoulder or sternum and may resemble that of angina or myocardial infarction – **refer**.

Pulmonary embolism
Pulmonary embolism is caused by a thrombus which has formed elsewhere and has detached itself from its primary site (e.g. a deep vein in the calf of the leg) and has been carried by the circulation to the lung, where it lodges in the pulmonary artery. The arterial lumen is blocked, causing lung tissue supplied by the artery to die (pulmonary infarct). The clinical picture is one of sudden onset chest pain and some dyspnoea; there may be blood in the sputum. Cough is a minor feature – **refer**.

Tuberculosis
Tuberculosis is a disease of slow onset and symptoms are often mild in its early stages. The tubercle bacillus is spread by inhalation of airborne droplets from an infected person. Tuberculosis is common in developing countries but does also occur in the UK. It is often overlooked in the elderly because of its insidious onset and its resemblance to bronchitis and congestive heart failure. Symptoms include a persistent cough, blood in the sputum (not always), fever or night sweats and weight loss. People at risk include the elderly, those who have contact with known cases, immigrants (especially from India) and alcoholics – **refer**.

Upper respiratory tract infection
Cough is a common accompaniment to viral infections, such as the common cold and flu-like illnesses. Irritation of the larynx and trachea by upper respiratory infection or a postnasal drip can cause a cough. The condition is generally self-limiting.

(continued overleaf)

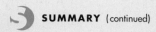 **SUMMARY** (continued)

Whooping cough

Although rare now because of immunisation programmes, whooping cough does still occur in children, usually under five years of age. The condition may present initially as a cold, and after a few days a cough develops, occurring at around hourly intervals. After about a week a whoop is heard on inspiration following a spasm of explosive coughing. The cough produces a plug of thick sputum, and is accompanied sometimes by vomiting. The patient will be frightened and distressed. The whoop may last for several weeks or months – **refer**.

Miscellaneous

Various relatively rare lung diseases are worth mentioning to highlight some of the possible causes that pharmacists should be alert to.

Fibrosing alveolitis is a chronic disease that causes reduced lung function, dyspnoea and cough. It is often autoimmune in origin. Rarely it may be due to drugs, the most commonly implicated compound being amiodarone. Nitrofurantoin and cytotoxic drugs have also been reported to cause the condition – **refer**.

Bird fancier's lung and farmer's lung are allergic conditions caused by inhalation of a protein in bird droppings (e.g. from racing pigeons) or of spores of a mould found in stored hay. Again, the picture is one of reduced lung function and cough – **refer**.

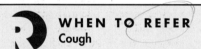 **WHEN TO REFER**
Cough

- Wheezing
- Dry night-time cough in children
- Difficulty in breathing, shortness of breath, breathlessness
- Any concurrent illness or history where infection may be a risk, depending on the severity of symptoms, e.g. chronic respiratory conditions, heart failure or immunosuppression
- Recurrent cough or constant smoker's cough, except where the doctor has given specific guidance for action to the patient at a previous consultation
- Chest pain, either uni- or bilateral, particularly if exacerbated on coughing or deep inspiration
- Sputum is purulent, i.e. unusual colour (green, brown) or foul smelling[*]
- Sputum is blood stained
- Concurrent medication includes ACE inhibitors
- Weight loss, particularly in patients over 40 years of age
- Painful or red, inflamed calf
- General malaise, feeling systemically unwell, persisting sweats or fever
- No improvement of symptoms after 7–14 days, depending on severity, or a deterioration in the condition with time

[*] Note that green sputum is commonly present in viral infections and may sometimes not justify referral, provided there are no other referable signs or symptoms. Purulent post-nasal drip may also be mistaken for sputum, which would not normally require referral.

CASE STUDIES

Case 1

A man in his mid 50s is well known to his pharmacist. Although not a frequent visitor he usually comes in two or three times each winter with a prescription for antibiotics, and has had at least two tries with nicotine replacement therapy. He has a heavy industrial occupation in a dusty factory where smoking is common, which probably does nothing to improve his health.

On this occasion he appears about two weeks after being treated for a chest infection, much improved but still coughing. The cough is no longer productive, but sounds moist and 'rattly', and he feels there is still 'something down there'. He asks for a bottle of linctus.

The pharmacist feels an expectorant to be most suitable, and it is duly supplied. However, there is considerable alarm a few days later when the man returns, holding his chest and complaining of a left-sided chest pain on breathing that is acute on coughing. He requests an analgesic but is easily persuaded to book in to the evening emergency surgery.

Relief is apparent early the following week, when he reappears feeling and looking better. A chest X-ray is normal, and an intercostal muscle strain the culprit, aggravated by the cough. To both their amusement he leaves with a starter pack of the latest television advertised nicotine treatment, but insists he is now determined. Apparently it was not only the cough that was rattled.

Case 2

The pharmacist usually finds time to pass the time of day with an elderly woman, in her late 70s, when she collects her prescription for a topical anti-inflammatory cream and a small dose of digoxin for her atrial fibrillation. A few weeks ago, she was anticoagulated, as a precursor to cardioversion, but persistent haemoptysis persuaded her doctors to forgo this in favour of a rather more holistic approach.

Now she has a cold, like many about her, with an irritating dry cough and a slight wheeze. It is not enough to keep her in, but certainly sufficient to interfere with sleep. A sympathomimetic bronchodilator seems appropriate.

Two days later she re-visits, suggesting that this medicine has made her short of breath. She is reassured that this is unlikely, but is clearly breathless on walking and is referred to her doctor without delay. She is seen quickly and returns with a prescription for a small quantity of bendrofluazide (bendroflumethiazide). It transpires, as often happens in this age group, that the infection has not itself progressed, but that it has produced a degree of heart failure and pulmonary oedema. Two weeks of treatment with the diuretic restored her to health.

Case 3

A fit 25-year-old man comes into the pharmacy. 'Nothing serious', he explains, meaning that it is nothing to worry his doctor about. Although he has a sedentary job, he plays a lot of sport and works out, and prides himself on his health. He thinks he has hay fever, the season being appropriate, and the symptoms are of rhinitis, a little wheeze on exertion and a fever.

The pharmacist is less convinced. The man does not look well, and is in some discomfort. He has in fact been febrile for two days, with an upper respiratory infection at first but now an increasingly painful dry cough, with pain on inspiration and movement, and breathlessness on minimal exertion. The possibilities are considered and reluctantly he accepts that even the fittest will occasionally succumb to illness and that there is no weakness in this.

He returns later that day from his doctor's walk-in clinic with a prescription for a potent antibiotic, a certificate for work for two weeks, and an appointment for follow up the next morning. He has an acute bronchitis, which could easily have taken him to hospital had he not recognised the signs and contacted his doctor so promptly. Yes, the pharmacist agrees, that was indeed fortunate.

4

Sore throats and colds

Conventionally, although somewhat arbitrarily, the respiratory system is divided into an upper part and a lower part. For practical purposes, the lower respiratory system can be considered as comprising the lungs, the bronchial tree and associated tissues, and the upper respiratory system comprises the larynx and all tissues above it. Thus, a cough is essentially a lower respiratory problem while head colds and sore throats are upper respiratory disorders.

Colds and sore throats, which often occur together, are common and are usually caused by viral infections. The major symptoms under consideration are sore throat, nasal congestion, catarrh, sneezing and rhinorrhoea (runny nose).

Sore throat

Assessing symptoms

Severity

A sore throat is generally a self-limiting condition.

Examining the back of the throat by asking the patient to open the mouth as wide as possible and then stick out the tongue will reveal on each side of the throat the anterior and posterior pillars of the fauces, between which the tonsils are situated (Figure 4.1). It is not possible to distinguish between the appearance of a viral infection and a bacterial infection, although it is thought that at least 70 per cent of sore throats are caused by viruses and are therefore not suitable for treatment with antibiotics.

If the soft palate, fauces and tonsils are very red or swollen and there are white spots of pus on the tonsils (Figure 4.2) or fauces, the patient should be referred. The pus spots may be a sign of streptococcal infection, which could respond to penicillin therapy.

The appearance of large, tender lymph nodes in the neck (see Figure 4.3) also requires a referral for the doctor to make a decision about the need for antibiotics.

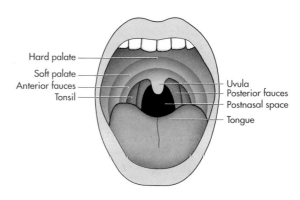

Figure 4.1 Diagram showing the position of the tonsils.

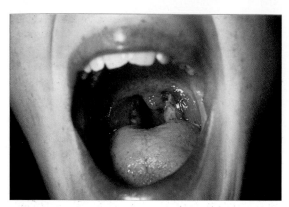

Figure 4.2   White spots of pus on enlarged tonsils.
(Reproduced with permission from Dr P. Marazzi/Science Photo Library.)

Difficulty in swallowing food or drink requires referral (see Accompanying symptoms).

It is worth pointing out that antibiotics were introduced into general practice between the two world wars at a time when severe conditions such as quinsy (peritonsillar abscess), mastoiditis (infection of the mastoid air cells in the middle ear) and rheumatic fever were all common. Widespread antibiotic use, and public health measures, caused the incidence of these three conditions to decline to the state of extreme rarity which is seen today. Thus, severe sequelae to sore throats are now so rare that the value of antibiotics is questionable, especially since in most cases the cause is viral. Without a throat swab to confirm whether the cause is viral or bacterial, prescribing decisions are made on subjective criteria, which will vary from one doctor to another. The medical profession is being urged to reduce the prescribing of antibiotics for upper respiratory tract infections. The severity of the discomfort, duration of the present condition and of past episodes, systemic upset and appearance of the pharynx may all be influential both for the doctor in prescribing and for the pharmacist in referring.

Duration and frequency

Sore throats caused by either viral or bacterial infections will usually disappear spontaneously within a few days, and as such they are not seri-ous. A sore throat persisting for more than one week should be referred. In teenagers and young adults, a persistent or recurrent sore throat requires referral to exclude glandular fever.

Recurrent sore throats should alert the pharmacist to various possible, but rare, causes such as immunosuppression caused by steroids (oral or inhaled) or by AIDS. Sore throat caused by drug deposition during inhalation of steroids can be reduced by advising the patient to rinse the mouth and gargle with water after inhaling.

Patients with undiagnosed or poorly controlled diabetes are susceptible to throat infections, especially those caused by fungi and yeasts, such as *Candida* (thrush). Oral thrush may be recognised by the appearance of white spots on the buccal mucosa and soft palate.

Patients should also be asked if they are taking any drugs, since some drugs can cause bone marrow suppression, resulting in a deficiency of white blood cells and repeated infections of the throat and other organs. These drugs include carbimazole, cytotoxic drugs, gold salts, tolbutamide, chlorpropamide, phenothiazines, antimalarials and some antibiotics. Patients taking these drugs should be referred urgently as the consequences of a lowered white cell count can be extremely serious.

Accompanying symptoms

Common cold

If symptoms of a cold are either already present or developing, it is likely that the sore throat is part of the cold syndrome, caused by a viral infection. For assessment of these symptoms, see below.

Difficulty in swallowing (dysphagia)

Anyone with a sore throat will find it less easy than normal to swallow, but if there is more than the expected degree of difficulty, then a referral should be considered. In children and teenagers with throat infections, especially tonsillitis, a sensation may develop of the throat 'closing over'. This is usually more apparent than real, but if drinking becomes very difficult or saliva cannot be swallowed, referral is advised. In extreme cases, such as quinsy, where there is an abscess on the tonsils, inflammation at the back of the throat may be so severe as potentially to restrict breathing. In very rare cases, dysphagia may be related to an obstruction in the throat or a tumour pressing on the oesophagus. It should be remembered that the reason for asking patients about difficulty in swallowing is to exclude those rare, severe cases where either the pharynx is dangerously inflamed or there is additional pathology causing obstruction which needs a medical opinion. It is often difficult to distinguish between a genuine difficulty in swallowing (dysphagia) and pain on swallowing. The latter can be expected with a sore throat and will be commonly complained of. Dysphagia, however, will be rarely encountered and apart from indicating a problem in the pharynx could also suggest a possible obstruction in the oesophagus caused, for instance, by a tumour. A pertinent question to ask is whether the patient can swallow liquids. If the answer is negative, then a referral should definitely be made.

Swollen lymph glands

Severe sore throats may be accompanied by swollen lymph glands in the neck (Figure 4.3). Referral is appropriate if the glands are extraordinarily painful or are not improving after five to seven days.

Earache

Infection in the pharynx can easily spread to the ear via the eustachian tube. Earache should be

referred if it has not improved after 48 hours or there is a discharge, since it is not only unpleasant for the patient but it may be caused by bacterial infection, which could be assessed for suitability for treatment with antibiotics.

Fever

A raised temperature may be a common accompaniment to a viral or bacterial throat infection and as such is of no great significance. However, patients with a persistent sore throat, especially with enlarged nodes in the neck, who complain of heavy sweats at night should be advised to see the doctor for a check up, since in rare cases this might reflect a neoplastic disease such as lymphoma. A high temperature in children raises the rare possibility of a convulsion and so should be treated. It is a sudden rise in temperature rather than a persistently elevated temperature that is thought to cause convulsions.

Hoarseness

Rather like dysphagia, some degree of hoarseness is to be expected with a sore throat, particularly when the larynx is involved. Laryngitis that does not resolve within five days requires a medical opinion regarding the value of starting antibiotics. Persistent and unusually severe hoarseness requires referral to exclude the possibility of any sinister cause.

Mouth ulceration

If a patient with a sore throat has ulcers or small petechial haemorrhages (purple or red spots) on the palate or the mucosa of the mouth, or ulcers and blistering on the lips and inside the mouth (Figure 4.4) an urgent medical opinion is required, especially if the patient is taking any of the drugs mentioned above (see Duration and frequency) as these are common symptoms of drug-induced bone marrow suppression.

The throat may also become ulcerated in the acute stage of glandular fever and in patients with aphthous (mouth) ulcers.

Rare causes of mouth ulceration include hand, foot and mouth disease (an infection unrelated to the bovine form with a similar name), mostly

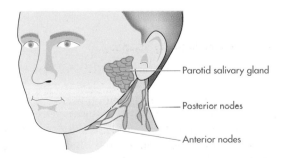

Figure 4.3 Main group of lymph nodes in the neck.

Parotid salivary gland

Posterior nodes

Anterior nodes

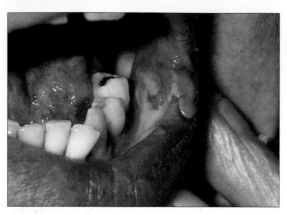

Figure 4.4   Mouth ulcer on the inside lower lip.
(Reproduced with permission from Dr P. Marazzi/Science Photo Library.)

seen in children, which produces a vesicular eruption at these sites only, is self-limiting and usually occurs in small epidemics. Also rare is Vincent's angina, another condition with a confusing name, in which a spirochaete infection produces ulcers on the gums and palate. This condition responds to treatment with metronidazole.

Myalgia (aches and pains)

Myalgia is common in patients with viral infections such as colds or flu and, unless persistent, it is of no consequence provided that the patient feels relatively well.

Severe malaise

Viral infections cause patients to feel ill and run down, but if there is severe malaise, particularly in the presence of other symptoms, then patients should be referred without delay.

Skin rash

A sore throat and a skin rash occurring together may reflect a reaction to a drug and, if suspected, the patient requires referral. Patients with glandular fever who have been treated with ampicillin or amoxicillin may develop a florid, itching rash all over the body, either during or shortly after finishing the course of antibiotic. Penicillin V should normally be the antibiotic of choice for streptococcal sore throats.

Special considerations

Patients with a history of endocarditis, rheumatic fever or those with artificial heart valves require special care, which usually includes antibiotic cover, when they have sore throats. This is because streptococcal infections can reach the heart valves and cause heart infection in these susceptible patients. A similar situation can arise in patients with a history of nephritis, who are susceptible to kidney infection.

These patients require medical attention.

Head cold

Assessing symptoms

The common cold (also called infectious rhinitis or acute coryza) presents with the well-known symptoms outlined below.

Congestion, rhinorrhoea and sneezing

Congestion

Nasal congestion is the most unpleasant and inconvenient symptom of the common cold. Excess mucus, particularly if it is purulent, suggests infection. In allergic rhinitis, the mucus will probably be clear and watery; this may also be the case, at least initially, in a patient with the common cold. Nasal congestion can be caused by some drugs, in particular antihypertensive agents which inhibit the sympathetic nervous system (e.g. alpha- and beta-blocking drugs) and oral contraceptives. Excess mucus may or may not be a feature.

Rhinorrhoea

Rhinorrhoea (runny nose) is a symptom of a cold as well as of allergic rhinitis. It often accompanies nasal congestion and is thought to result from the engorgement of the nasal mucosa with blood, which narrows the lumen of the nasal passages and also stimulates the mucus-secreting glands in the mucosa.

Sneezing

Sneezing may occur in the common cold and also in allergic rhinitis. In allergic rhinitis, sneezing is likely to be paroxysmal (occurring as a bout or fit of repetitive sneezing) and accompanied by itchiness in the nose. These characteristics help to distinguish an allergic cause from a viral infection.

Onset and duration

The common cold normally lasts for a few days and not longer than two weeks. Symptoms beyond this time should be reassessed, bearing in mind the possibility of allergic rhinitis. In the summer months this is most likely to be caused by pollen allergy (hay fever). Ninety per cent of UK hay fever sufferers are allergic to grass pollen (most prolific in May and June) and 25 per cent have an allergy to tree pollen (April to May). At other times of the year allergy may be due to hypersensitivity to antigens found in dust, the spores of some fungi, animal dander, feathers and other materials in the home or workplace. This type of allergy, which may persist throughout the year, is termed perennial rhinitis. It produces symptoms continuously or in irregular episodes when the concentration of allergen in the atmosphere is particularly high.

Accompanying symptoms

Nasal symptoms are often accompanied by shivering, sweating, headaches, sore throats and sometimes earache, the latter especially in children.

Conjunctivitis

Red eyes may be a sign of a common viral infection such as the common cold but are better known as an accompaniment to allergic rhinitis. In allergic rhinitis, the eyes usually itch and the patient will rub them, whereas in the common cold this is not a predominant feature. Patients with allergic rhinitis often also complain of an itchy palate; this sometimes occurs before the nose and eye symptoms develop.

Myalgia

Aching muscles and joints accompany a viral respiratory infection, when the diagnosis is often known as flu or influenza.

Cough

The common cold often spreads to the lower respiratory tract and a cough may then result. Symptoms should be assessed according to the guidelines given on cough described in Chapter 3.

Sinusitis

Tender sinuses, headache, dizziness or a feeling of fullness in the head, together with purulent mucus, may be a sign of sinusitis (see Chapter 2).

Special considerations in children

Upper respiratory infections are at least as common in children as in adults. The chronic catarrhal child syndrome occurs in children aged between four and eight years and results in recurrent colds, from which there seems to be no respite. It is helpful to reassure the parents that the episode will be self-limiting, and that the child will grow out of the condition. If the condition is severe, particularly with frequent ear infections or suspected deafness, the child should be referred.

In teenagers with sore throats the possibility of glandular fever should be considered if the sore throat is persistent and the patient feels ill.

In younger children, recurrent tonsillitis may require tonsillectomy. Inflammation of the adenoids (or pharyngeal tonsils), which are lymph nodes lying in the nasopharynx, causes adenoiditis and this frequently accompanies tonsillitis in children. The adenoids may become enlarged as a result of normal growth as well as from inflammation and, in either case, can cause nasal obstruction or blockage of the eustachian tubes. Symptoms include mouth breathing, snoring during sleep and ear infections. Referral is necessary in recurrent cases to consider surgical removal of the adenoids.

Upper respiratory tract symptoms often herald the onset of the childhood infectious diseases, such as chickenpox, and parents should be advised to look out for the appearance of a rash.

Babies who are teething often suffer from the symptoms of upper respiratory tract disease. These are usually short lived and can be treated symptomatically with paediatric paracetamol syrup.

Management

The traditional advice to sufferers of the common cold is to take some aspirin or paracetamol, keep warm and drink plenty of fluids. This is generally sound advice in that the best approach is to provide symptomatic relief. There are also many proprietary products marketed for symptom relief.

NB: Aspirin should not be given to children under 12 years.

Fluid intake and steam inhalations

A high fluid intake maintains adequate hydration of the body to counteract excessive fluid loss caused by fever. It also increases hydration of the mucous membranes. Steam inhalations provide local hydration of the tissues of the upper respiratory tract and dilute the secretion of mucus, making it less viscous and tenacious.

Decongestants

Oral sympathomimetic agents

Nasal congestion in the common cold is caused by an inflammatory reaction in the lining of the nose, causing dilatation and engorgement of blood vessels and oedema of the mucous membranes.

Stimulation of alpha-adrenoceptors causes vasoconstriction in the nasal mucosa, resulting in a shrinkage of the inflamed tissue and an increase in the lumen of the nasal passages, facilitating breathing and drainage of mucus. The most commonly used decongestant sympathomimetic drugs in oral preparations are phenylpropanolamine, phenylephrine, ephedrine and pseudoephedrine.

Studies have shown that phenylpropanolamine in particular can increase the blood pressure of young, healthy people, although this has generally been in doses above those recommended for use as a decongestant. Sustained-release preparations are thought to be less of a problem in this respect than conventional-release products. While it may be assumed that there will be no significant clinical sequelae in normotensive patients taking recommended doses, the products should be avoided in hypertensive patients and in patients with ischaemic heart disease because of the adverse consequences of pressor effects.

Sympathomimetics are also contraindicated in patients taking monoamine oxidase inhibitors and those with hyperthyroidism. Because of their beta-agonist activity, these agents may disturb blood glucose control by an anti-insulin effect and hence they are best avoided by diabetic patients. If a sympathomimetic agent is requested by a patient in one of these categories, locally acting formulations, such as nasal drops or spray, should be recommended so that any possible systemic effects are kept to a minimum.

Sympathomimetic amines also have bronchodilator effects through stimulation of beta-receptors and are commonly found in combination remedies for coughs and colds.

Oral decongestants are rarely found as the sole active principle in OTC products. The contents of some typical products are shown in Table 4.1. Their interactions with prescribed drugs are given in Table 4.2.

Nasal sprays and drops

Sympathomimetic agents provide rapid and effective relief from nasal congestion when applied locally to the nasal membranes. The most commonly used are ephedrine, phenylephrine and naphazoline, which are relatively short acting, and oxymetazolone and xylometazolone, which are claimed to have a duration of action of up to eight hours.

Local decongestants produce relatively few systemic side effects because the local vasocon-striction reduces drug absorption from the site of application.

The use of local decongestants is associated with a phenomenon known as rhinitis medicamentosa. This is a rebound effect in which congestion follows the vasoconstrictive effect. The longer-acting agents are reputedly less likely to cause this effect, although the evidence for this is poor. The phenomenon can be avoided by reducing usage to no more than seven days.

Antihistamines

Antihistamines are effective in colds and allergic rhinitis because of their intrinsic anticholinergic properties. The drugs suppress the production of mucus in the nasal mucosa and thus give symptomatic relief in rhinorrhoea, as well as reducing the postnasal drip that irritates the pharynx and causes coughing. Traditional antihistamines are

Table 4.1 Examples of combination cold remedies

Sympathomimetic	Antihistamine	Other constituents
Pseudoephedrine		Paracetamol
Pseudoephedrine	Triprolidine	
Phenylpropanolamine		Paracetamol, ipecacuanha
Phenylephrine and phenylpropanolamine	Brompheniramine	
Phenylpropanolamine	Chlorpheniramine (chlorphenamine)	
Phenylpropanolamine	Chlorpheniramine (chlorphenamine)	Dextromethorphan, paracetamol

Table 4.2 Interactions between OTC products for colds and prescribed drugs

OTC product	Interacting drug	Consequence
Antihistamines	CNS sedatives	Enhanced sedation
	Anticholinergic drugs, including tricyclic antidepressants	Enhanced anticholinergic effect, e.g. dry mouth, blurred vision, constipation and urinary retention
Sympathomimetics (particularly oral formulations)	Antihypertensive drugs	Reduced antihypertensive effects
	MAOIs	Hypertensive crisis
	Tricyclic antidepressants	Hypertension possible with phenylephrine (less likely with ephedrine and phenylpropanolamine)

well known for their sedative effects but the more recently introduced ones, such as loratadine, cetirizine and acrivastine, are less likely to cause sedation. Because of their anticholinergic effects, antihistamines should not be recommended to patients with narrow-angle glaucoma or prostatism. They can also cause dry mouth, constipation and palpitations, and can interfere with accommodation in the eye in some patients.

Eye-drops containing antihistamines can help to provide rapid alleviation of itchy conjunctivitis in hay fever.

Cromoglicate

Sodium cromoglicate nasal preparations are available for prophylaxis in hay fever and, like intranasal steroids, should be used continuously.

Intranasal steroids

Nasal sprays containing steroids such as beclometasone and flunisolide reduce nasal congestion in seasonal allergic rhinitis (hay fever) by a local anti-inflammatory effect. They may take several days to exert maximum effect and should be used regularly throughout the season as a prophylactic measure.

Lozenges

Lozenges have a traditional place in the treatment of sore throats. However, the clinical benefit of antibacterial agents is tenuous, especially given that many sore throats are caused by viruses. The most useful effect of lozenges lies in their ability to stimulate the flow of saliva, which acts as a demulcent and soothes the pharynx. Many lozenges contain benzocaine, but the amount is probably too small to offer any real benefit.

Zinc

The results of some clinical studies have suggested that zinc lozenges (containing approximately 13 to 23 mg zinc) may have a beneficial effect in the common cold by reducing both the severity and duration of symptoms. It is believed that zinc ions combine with the rhinovirus coating to prevent the virus entering cells and reproducing further. It is recommended that one lozenge is sucked every two hours, commencing at the earliest sign of symptoms. It is unclear whether tablets containing zinc salts will have the same beneficial effect as that attributed to the lozenges.

Menthol

Menthol and other oils, such as eucalyptus, are present in many formulations that alleviate the symptoms of the common cold. These include inhalations, pastilles and nasal sprays. As well as having a great placebo effect, these oils do appear to relieve nasal congestion. They should not be used regularly for long periods as they may damage the cilia in the respiratory mucosa.

Vitamin C

Vitamin C is the best-known prophylactic agent for the common cold, but its efficacy is controversial. It is of interest to note that Linus Pauling, the great protagonist for its use, stated that doses of about 3 g per day were necessary for prophylaxis and 1 or 2 g per hour is required to suppress symptoms when they appear.

SUMMARY OF CONDITIONS PRODUCING SORE THROATS AND COLDS

Allergic rhinitis

Allergic rhinitis may be seasonal (as in hay fever) or perennial. It is caused by sensitivity to various components in the atmosphere, such as pollen, dust and pollutants. The main symptoms are itchy nose, sneezing, rhinorrhoea and red, itching eyes.

Glandular fever

Glandular fever (infectious mononucleosis) presents as a persistent, severe sore throat in a teenager or young adult and is accompanied by enlarged, tender lymph glands, either in the neck or elsewhere. The patient feels ill and weak. The first attack will resolve in two to four weeks, but the condition recurs, each subsequent attack being after a longer time and milder than the last. The process can take several months, rarely up to two years, and the fatigue persists between attacks. It is important to rest when feeling ill, both to shorten the illness and to guard against the development of post-viral syndrome. The diagnosis can be confirmed by a blood test – **refer**.

Influenza

Influenza is a viral infection which produces upper and sometimes also lower respiratory symptoms accompanied by systemic symptoms such as malaise, myalgia (aching muscles) and fever. True influenza can only be diagnosed during epidemics and confirmation of an epidemic is given by public health teams. In the absence of this official label, the majority of such cases are labelled 'flu-like'. The distinction clinically can be less clear. At-risk groups such as the elderly and patients with chronic diseases, especially respiratory conditions but also cardiovascular disease and diabetes, should be advised to inquire from their local medical practice about their suitability for vaccination against influenza.

Laryngitis

Laryngitis is inflammation of the larynx (voice box) characterised by hoarseness. It may be a complication of an upper respiratory infection, such as a cold or sore throat, or may be caused by the inhalation of irritants, such as tobacco smoke. If present for more than a few days, antibiotic treatment may be considered. If persistent for longer periods and accompanied by difficulty in swallowing, more sinister but rarer causes such as laryngeal or pharyngeal tumours should be excluded – **refer** if persistent.

Tonsillitis

Tonsillitis is an acute inflammation of the palatine tonsils caused by bacterial or viral infection. The tonsils appear red and swollen, sometimes with white flecks of pus. The result may be difficulty in swallowing and the neck glands may be tender and enlarged – refer if there is no improvement after three days.

Quinsy is an abscess on the tonsils. It is a rare condition that may develop about one week after the onset of tonsillitis. The throat is painful and pain may spread to the ear. The patient feels ill and there is difficulty in swallowing and some obstruction to breathing – **refer**.

Adenoiditis occurs principally in children and may accompany tonsillitis (see above).

Thrush

Thrush (candidiasis) can cause sore throats. In adults, it is more common in the elderly (especially those with ill-fitting dentures) and in patients taking steroids (oral or inhaled) or other immunosuppressive drugs or antibiotics. It may resolve spontaneously – **refer** if persistent.

WHEN TO REFER

Sore throats and colds

Sore throats
- Tonsils red and swollen with pus or white spots visible
- Accompanied by ulcers on palate or buccal mucosa
- Concurrent drugs include carbimazole, phenothiazines, antibiotics, cytotoxic drugs, gold and chlorpropamide
- Patient is immunosuppressed or taking steroids
- Accompanied by skin rash
- History of endocarditis, rheumatic fever or artificial heart valves
- Accompanied by painful enlarged lymph glands in the neck, or enlarged glands that do not improve within five to seven days
- Long-term or recurrent hoarseness or loss of voice
- Earache that does not resolve after 48 hours or is accompanied by a discharge
- Difficulty in swallowing
- Recurrent tonsillitis in children

Colds
- Purulent mucus for several days
- Sinus or ear pain that does not resolve after seven days
- Difficulty in breathing
- Wheezing, especially in young children
- Malaise in teenagers and young adults for more than seven days
- Severe symptoms that do not improve within seven days

CASE STUDIES

Case 1

One Saturday afternoon a man in his late 20s comes into the pharmacy, and asks to speak to the pharmacist. He is smartly and fashionably dressed.

He has had a sore throat with catarrh and a cough for almost a week. He has heard from the media of the advice to take such problems to a pharmacist, but has an important and busy job, and cannot afford any time off work. Antibiotics were clearly the solution, but after waiting three days to see his doctor he was told not only that they would have no effect, but that evidence had proved cough and cold remedies to be of no clinical value, and he had no alternative but to 'ride it out'.

This is a difficult, but increasingly common, problem for pharmacists, and the pharmacist patiently explains the nature of these infections. The vast majority, the pharmacist agrees, are viral in nature, and the patient's history is suggestive of this. Antibiotics have therefore no useful role. Reluctantly agreeing, the young man gestures to the impressive display of proprietary remedies and adds that if there is no cure, perhaps all these medicines are no more than a means of duping the unsuspecting public.

→

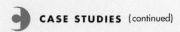

CASE STUDIES (continued)

The pharmacist agrees with the doctor that nothing can be recommended that will influence the course or duration of the illness, but the pharmacist can use his experience to find something for symptomatic relief. For a man whose concern is to continue his work uninterrupted, surely this is of some value. The appropriate questions are asked and a product selected.

Time passes and the customer is not seen again. Whether he was convinced, and whether the medication worked the pharmacist will never know, but wisely chooses to believe that it did.

Case 2

A man in his mid 30s is seen in the pharmacy, requesting help with a sore throat. He is otherwise well, and a recommendation is made.

He returns, however, about six weeks later. Another sore throat, but rather worse this time, with some systemic disturbance of fever, myalgia and tiredness. He was in two minds about seeing his doctor, but the medicine before was effective and he thought he would try that again first. The pharmacist is less certain, and recommends he consult his doctor.

Although he has no obvious tonsillitis, with no exudate in his throat, he does have cervical adenitis and returns with a prescription for antibiotics. The pharmacist is encouraged by the thought that this doctor too hedges his or her bets when unsure.

After another month the man is back again, with more antibiotics. The infection did not completely resolve, and in particular the glands never subsided. Progressively the general malaise has increased, and his doctor is also investigating this with blood tests.

Finally he returns once more, this time with a prescription for analgesics. He has lost weight and looks visibly ill. The blood count was abnormal, and a scan following the discovery of an enlarged spleen suggested a lymphoma. A biopsy of one of the glands confirms Hodgkin's disease, a neoplasm of the lymphoid system characterised by chronic enlargement of the lymph nodes, with enlargement of the spleen and often of the liver, and often anemia and recurring fevers. The patient is now going into hospital for staging and treatment, and as he leaves the shop the pharmacist is left with a profound sense of sorrow, but also the concern that the diagnosis might have been made earlier. Unfortunately there are many insidious presentations in medicine where the underlying diagnosis is often delayed, and where all pharmacists can do is to try to maintain a high index of suspicion; that is, never assume that because common problems are frequently seen, rarer ones will not occasionally appear.

Case 3

This woman is well known to her pharmacist. She has three young children and visited fairly often during her pregnancies, and afterwards with prescriptions for the children's minor ailments.

The youngest child, now almost a year old, has been the most difficult. Her doctor, health visitor and the pharmacist have treated several episodes of 'snuffles', or nasal congestion, with only limited success. She complains the child has always been a poor feeder, and a variety of artificial milks were recommended, including changing to a soya-based preparation for a time. The recurrent catarrhal problems seem to have continued unabated. They are often considered to be colds or flu, with requests for antibiotics. These have been tried on one or two occasions, but, like the other remedies, with little or no effect. The problem has been complicated by one more serious problem, a chest infection that necessitated admission to hospital and reinforced in everybody's minds the need for vigilance.

Even now the child eats poorly and unhealthily, and is frequently seen with colds, coughs and earache.

(continued overleaf)

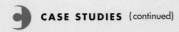

CASE STUDIES (continued)

This is a common problem that is distressing for all concerned, as it can be very difficult to unravel often multiple causes. Diet is often blamed for catarrhal problems in early life, perhaps because other possibilities seem less convincing. Infection is obviously important, usually repeated and low grade, and maybe associated with immunological difficulties. Younger children may be exposed early to infections brought home by their older siblings, but the evidence for all of this is hard to find.

Clearly what is required is sensible and practical advice that is realistic in its objectives without offering false reassurance. Equally it is vital that the professionals involved do not contradict each other. In this case the health visitor, who visited the pharmacy frequently herself, obtained consent to discuss the child both with the doctor and pharmacist. They agreed that on many occasions the child appeared well and adequately nourished, and that reassurance for a busy and harassed mother with practical symptomatic relief was the most important message. At the same time, she should not be dismissed as 'inadequate' or hypochondriacal, for occasional ear and other infections were happening which needed intervention.

With time the condition most commonly improves, as it did in this instance, although there is the prospect that it will continue as a chronic catarrhal state requiring a specialist opinion and perhaps a minor surgical procedure such as the insertion of grommets into the ears or, less frequently now, adenoidectomy.

5

Eye disorders

Because of the emotive overtones surrounding diseases of the eye, some pharmacists may consider it inappropriate to treat any condition affecting the eye. However, by following the normal protocol to establish the history of the disorder and applying some common sense, it is relatively easy to decide whether a medical referral is necessary.

Types of eye disorders

Generally, the eye conditions presenting to pharmacists will be disorders either of the eyeball itself or of the eyelids. These can be broadly classified as:

1. The painless red eye
2. Inflammation of the eyelids
3. Disorders of tear formation or drainage
4. The painful eye
5. Eye disorders which are a manifestation of a more generalised disease.

Foreign bodies in the eye requiring first aid treatment will not be considered here.

The first three categories are relatively easy to recognise, usually present no immediate danger to the patient and in most cases can be treated symptomatically in the first instance. The painful eye requires referral and patients will generally need to see a doctor reasonably urgently, according to severity. Diseases in the fifth category will usually manifest themselves with unusual signs or symptoms, so that it will be obvious to an intelligent observer that something serious is wrong. Proptosis (exophthalmos), which is the bulging of the eyes

from the sockets, is common in patients with an overactive thyroid gland. Bulging of one eye, however, raises the possibility of some local pathology behind the eye and requires investigation.

Blurred vision or double vision may be a sign of early demyelinating disease, such as multiple sclerosis, or of a tumour in the brain. Nystagmus, which describes the continuous movement of the eye in a horizontal or vertical direction, may indicate some brain disorder. Nystagmus is also a sign of phenytoin toxicity, when serum levels of the drug exceed the therapeutic range. These types of more serious disease will be seen relatively rarely in the pharmacy.

The rest of this chapter will show how to differentiate major and minor disease in the first four categories listed above.

A diagrammatic representation of the eye is shown in Figure 5.1.

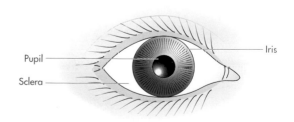

Figure 5.1 Anterior view of the eye.

Assessing symptoms

Site and type

Conjunctiva

Inflammation of the anterior eye (Figure 5.2) occurs in conjunctivitis. In both allergic and infective conjunctivitis, the white (sclera) of the eye is red and this redness extends to the inner surface of the eyelids (Figure 5.3).

Pulling down the lower lid will reveal a very red conjunctiva covering its inner surface compared with the pale pink colour which is seen in a normal eye.

If both eyes are affected and in the absence of any warning signs or symptoms the conjunctivitis will probably have either an allergic or an infective cause.

In allergic conjunctivitis, there will be no pus, but there is usually a watery discharge, which distinguishes it from the infective type. The commonest cause of allergic conjunctivitis is hay fever.

Allergic conjunctivitis is often seen in young people, in whom any allergic predispositions are

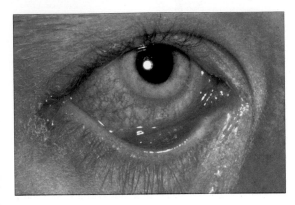

Figure 5.3   Conjunctivitis. (Reproduced with permission from St Bartholomew's Hospital/Science Photo Library.)

more evident. The patient is commonly female, and the cause is often eye cosmetics, although soaps, cleansers and powders applied to the face can also provoke a reaction.

Hypoallergenic preparations will still affect some people and the condition will only clear after total avoidance of cosmetics around the eyes.

Conjunctivitis commonly affects both eyes, although one may be affected more than the other. A unilateral red eye is more likely to be related to a condition within the eye, such as iritis (inflammation of the iris) or glaucoma. In such cases the redness typically occurs more around the centre of the eye, close to the iris, and is largely absent from inside the lids, as compared with the more peripheral redness of an allergy or infection. However, it is often difficult to distinguish the conditions on this basis.

In wearers of contact lenses, conjunctivitis can be caused by a scratched cornea, a reaction to a lens solution, a poorly fitting lens or corneal drying.

A subconjunctival haemorrhage, caused by a burst blood vessel, appears as a red spot on the white of the eye (Figure 5.4). Although it can provoke much anxiety in the sufferer, it is harmless and will heal spontaneously without treatment, provided that no accompanying symptoms are present.

Patients who complain of dry eyes may require artificial tears (as eye-drops). This condition is seen as a complication of certain disorders, such as rheumatoid arthritis (Sjögren's syndrome),

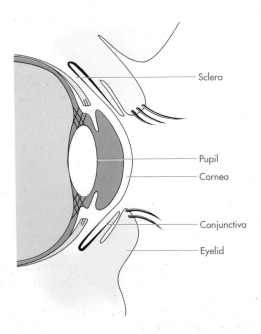

— Sclera

— Pupil

— Cornea

— Conjunctiva

— Eyelid

Figure 5.2   Horizontal cross-section of the anterior eye.

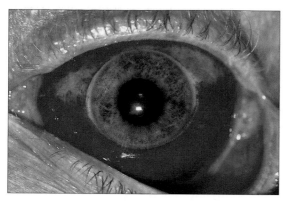

Figure 5.4 Subconjunctival haemorrhage. (Reproduced with permission from the Science Photo Library.)

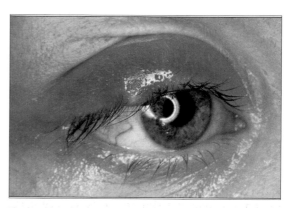

Figure 5.5 Stye on the upper eyelid. (Reproduced with permission from Western Ophthalmic Hospital/Science Photo Library.)

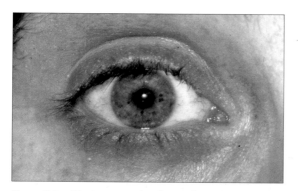

Figure 5.6 Blepharitis, with inflammation of the eyelid. (Reproduced with permission from Jane Shamilt Cosine Graphics/Science Photo Library.)

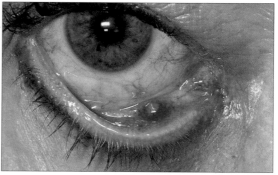

Figure 5.7 Meibomian cyst (chalazion). (Reproduced with permission from Dr P. Marazzi/Science Photo Library.)

and in oestrogen deficiency, as occurs in menopausal women. It is wise to refer patients with dry eyes to eliminate corneal ulceration or any other pathology.

Eyelids

Inflammation of the margin of one eyelid is likely to be caused by a small abscess or stye (an infection of a hair follicle gland at the base of an eyelash; Figure 5.5). The inflammation will be localised at first but may spread to involve the rest of the eyelid, which will become tender and painful. After one or two days the stye will usually come to a head and may burst or simply shrink and resolve. Those which do not resolve may require surgical excision.

Redness and irritation of the eyelid margins (affecting one or both eyes), often with scales adhering to the base of eyelashes, occurs in blepharitis (Figure 5.6). This is commonly associated with seborrhoeic dermatitis or dandruff, or it may be allergic, in which case concurrent conjunctivitis may also be noticed. More rarely, it may be caused by infection. Some eyelashes may be either absent or distorted, sometimes pointing inwards and irritating the surface of the eye. If the cause is infective, pus may be seen discharging from the base of the lashes.

Displacement of the eyelids may be seen, particularly in the elderly. In such cases, the margins of the eyelids do not close together when the eyes are closed. Spasm or atony of the orbital muscles causes the lids either to invert (entropion; see Figure 5.10) or to evert (ectropion; see

Figure 5.11). In the former case, the lid margins and lashes point inwards and irritate the eye, while in the latter the lower lids fall away from the eye, offering it insufficient protection and lubrication. In ectropion, the drainage of the tear film is deranged and tears roll down the face.

A hard pea-like lump appearing under the skin of the lid, most commonly the upper lid, away from the eyelid margin, will probably be a meibomian cyst (chalazion). They may also be found in the lower lid, visualised by pulling down the lower lid to reveal a small lump resembling an internal stye under the conjunctiva (Figure 5.7). This is an infection of one of the meibomian glands, which are located deep in the cartilaginous tissue on the underside of the lids and secrete fluid onto the conjunctiva. Infection of the outlet of a gland results in blockage and inflammation in the same way that a stye forms. The cyst will normally resolve spontaneously without incident but may recur from time to time in some patients. Any persistent cysts may require surgery.

A drooping upper eyelid (ptosis; Figure 5.8) is often a sign of systemic disease, such as myasthenia gravis, and referral is essential. In babies, special measures are needed to rectify the droop to avoid reduced visual input to the brain and blindness. Ptosis is also a sign of Horner's syndrome, which is caused by a lesion in the cervical sympathetic nerve, often due to trauma, tumours or bleeds.

Retraction of the eyelids may be a sign of a bulging eyeball, which is seen in patients with an overactive thyroid gland. In a mild form it is

difficult for the untrained observer to detect, but a gap of white sclera between the iris and the affected lid will be seen if the patient's eye is compared with a normal eye. The accompanying symptoms of thyrotoxicosis (see below) will alert the observer to the condition.

Intensity

It should be relatively easy to distinguish a superficial itching or irritation of the conjunctiva on the surface of the eye from a more intense pain caused by pathology within the eye itself. Any such pain, which may be accompanied by the other symptoms or signs described below, requires a medical opinion. If severe, referral should be made urgently.

Duration

Styes and bacterial conjunctivitis will normally resolve spontaneously within a few days and can be helped by OTC medicines.

Viral conjunctivitis may last for one to two weeks. There is no specific treatment and it will eventually resolve spontaneously. Patients should be told to report any worsening of symptoms or the appearance of pain or deterioration of vision as these may indicate a rare involvement of the cornea.

Meibomian cysts and subconjunctival haemorrhages may take a few weeks to disappear, but will do so without the need for treatment. Entropion and ectropion will usually have been present for a long time when brought to the attention of the pharmacist and will require no urgent treatment, although referral for a medical opinion may be appropriate if the patient is anxious or worried about the condition.

Blepharitis that has not responded to appropriate OTC remedies within seven days should be referred for treatment with antibiotic eye ointment, since delay may result in the condition becoming a chronic problem.

Any pain within the eye or any visual disturbance requires same-day referral to a doctor or hospital emergency department to exclude serious disease.

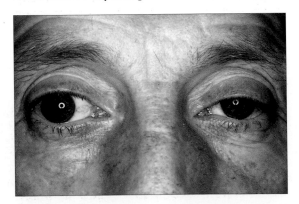

Figure 5.8 Ptosis. (Reproduced with permission from the Wellcome Trust Medical Photographic Library.)

Accompanying symptoms

Pain

Itchiness, grittiness and soreness felt on the surface of the eye are common symptoms of minor superficial conditions, such as conjunctivitis. These symptoms should be distinguished from a deep-seated pain arising from within the eye which indicates possible serious pathology, such as a raised intraocular pressure (glaucoma) or iritis, and requires urgent referral. Similarly, trauma such as flash burns (in welders working with oxyacetylene burners) and corneal injury will cause severe pain.

A feeling of grittiness on the surface of one eye will frequently be caused by a foreign body.

Nasal symptoms

Conjunctivitis accompanied by nasal symptoms, such as congestion, sneezing and rhinorrhoea, suggests an allergic component to the condition. A sore throat, symptoms of a cold or general malaise may be associated with a viral conjunctivitis, which is usually caused by an adenovirus.

Visual disturbance

A loss of vision is a medical emergency. Disturbance of vision may be due to the visual component of migraine, in which case it is likely to be recurrent and recognised by the patient. In conjunctivitis, vision is not significantly affected because the conjunctiva does not cover the cornea and the underlying pupil, and thus light enters and penetrates the eye in the normal manner. Vision may temporarily be affected if the cornea is obscured by fluid or pus. Loss of visual acuity is often accompanied by pain within the eye, but there are exceptions, such as vascular blockage or haemorrhages in the eye, optic nerve damage, temporal arteritis (see Chapter 2) or retinal detachment, which will not be painful.

Double vision accompanied by ptosis and a headache of sudden onset suggests the possibility of an intracranial bleed and requires urgent medical attention.

Bizarre patterns in the field of vision, with haloes seen around bright lights (particularly noticed when coming out of a dark into a lit area, e.g. when leaving a cinema, or driving at night), require referral as this is seen in glaucoma and multiple sclerosis (known as optic neuritis in the latter case). The patient should be advised to seek advice with the suspicion of multiple sclerosis left unstated, since the diagnosis may prove to be different and in any case requires careful handling by a clinician. The visual disturbances which accompany classical migraine are easily distinguishable from those described here (see Chapter 2).

Tired eyes

Complaints of tired and sore eyes may be associated with conjunctivitis; in the absence of this condition, a referral to the optometrist may be in order to check for eye strain and any defects in visual acuity.

Lacrimation

Lacrimation is associated with interrupted drainage of the tear film and in babies requires referral so that the condition can be rectified. In elderly patients it will be seen in ectropion.

Discharge

A discharge of pus which collects in the inner corner of the eye or which prevents easy opening of the eyelids on awakening is a sign of bacterial conjunctivitis. This may be unilateral but usually affects both eyes. A clear watery discharge occurs in allergic and viral conjunctivitis.

Pupils

It is wise to carry out a simple physical examination of the eyes, especially if a serious condition is suspected. The pupils should be round and of equal size. They should react equally and oppositely to light such that each will constrict when a light is directed at it. The pupil should remain circular as it constricts; irregularity suggests adhesions from iritis. (This may be a previously diagnosed condition and the patient should be questioned before assuming it is recent.) Any inequality or abnormality of size, shape or reaction will suggest serious pathology within the eye and the need for immediate referral.

A hazy or cloudy appearance to the iris or pupil may be caused by inflammatory exudate in the anterior chamber (as in iritis) or corneal oedema (as in glaucoma) and therefore requires medical referral.

Bulging eye

A rare presentation of a bulging eye (proptosis) or of retracted eyelids (upper, lower or both) may be accompanied by symptoms of an overactive thyroid such as sweating, hot skin, flushing, tremor of the hands or fingers, weight loss despite an increasing appetite, fast heart rate and a state of physical overactivity.

Headache

Headaches accompanying eye symptoms can occur in glaucoma, migraine and temporal arteritis. The nature of the headache will assist in differentiating these conditions.

Aggravating factors

Irritation by light (photophobia) may occur in many eye conditions, including conjunctivitis, corneal ulcers and iritis. Although not very helpful in differentiating eye conditions, its presence should be borne in mind as it is a feature of conditions such as meningitis and migraine.

Conjunctivitis may be aggravated by smoke, dust, pollen or cosmetics and in some instances these irritants will be the causative factors.

Special considerations: age

All babies under two months old should be referred. Babies with eyes that discharge pus may have specific infections acquired during birth that require appropriate diagnosis and prescription of antibiotics to prevent serious consequences.

Older babies commonly acquire infective conjunctivitis. In their mild forms these infections are of no consequence and can be treated symptomatically by simple measures, such as bathing the eyelid margins with clean water.

Ptosis in babies requires medical attention to keep the lid open. Failure to do so will result in a lack of visual stimulation to the retina and eventual blindness.

A squint in children requires correction to prevent a 'lazy eye', which after the age of about five years cannot be rectified.

Some eye conditions are more common in the elderly and should be borne in mind when assessing an older patient. In temporal arteritis the visual loss, which will be permanent, is preceded by headaches and temporal tenderness (see Chapter 2). Glaucoma has a greater incidence in the middle-aged and elderly population.

The lens of the eye gradually becomes more opaque with age, which can cause cataracts and visual loss in elderly patients. The cornea covering the pupil and iris becomes cloudy. Although cataracts do not require urgent medical attention, referral is necessary if there is any visual loss.

Subconjunctival haemorrhages, dry eyes, ectropion and entropion are all more common in the elderly.

Management

If an eye condition does not respond to appropriate simple self-medication within seven days, patients should usually be advised to seek medical advice. This is because some conditions may become chronic, for example blepharitis, and some may need antibiotics, for example severe infective conjunctivitis.

Antibacterial eye-drops and ointments

Propamidine and dibrompropamidine are active against the organisms that are commonly implicated in eye infections, such as staphylococci, streptococci and *Haemophilus influenzae* in bacterial conjunctivitis, and staphylococci in styes and infective blepharitis. The efficacy of propamidine eye-drops can probably be max-imised in the treatment of conjunctivitis by hourly instillation, at least for the first day of treatment. Eye ointment containing dibrompro-pamidine is suitable as a once or twice daily application to the eyelid margins in infective blepharitis and styes. Styes usually resolve spon-taneously without the application of antibacter-ial preparations. Failure to reduce symptoms within seven days requires referral to the doctor for assessment.

Scales or pus adhering to the lid margins can be loosened and lifted by the use of antibacterial eye ointment and by wiping the lid margins with diluted baby shampoo, which is unperfumed and non-irritant to the eyes.

Simple hygiene measures, such as the use of separate face flannels and towels, may be helpful in preventing the spread of infection to other family members.

Vasoconstrictor substances

Various sympathomimetic agents, such as phenylephrine, adrenaline (epinephrine), napha-zoline and xylometazoline, are present in OTC eye-drops. In conjunctivitis, these drugs reduce the injection of the conjunctiva with blood by a vasconstrictive action. They not only serve a cos-metic function but also reduce the irritation caused by the conjunctival hyperaemia and inflammation. They should not be used in patients with concurrent eye disease such as glaucoma.

Antihistamines

The cause of allergic conjunctivitis, such as pollen or cosmetics, should be identified and where possible removed. The use of eye-drops containing an antihistamine, such as antazoline, in combination with a vasoconstrictor drug is effective in providing symptomatic relief in this condition. If nasal symptoms are also present, as in allergic rhinitis, oral antihistamines should be recommended in addition to eye-drops.

Cromoglicate

Sodium cromoglicate eye-drops give sympto-matic relief of allergic conjunctivitis caused by hay fever.

Astringent eye lotions

Eye lotions that contain astringents such as witch hazel are promoted for treatment of irrita-tion and red eyes. They are best recommended where no specific syndrome exists, for example in cases where a patient complains of 'tired eyes' but has no significant conjunctivitis.

Other measures

A stye may be drawn to a point to facilitate exu-dation of pus by applying a hot compress to the lid. This can be done by soaking a clean towel or flannel in hot water and placing it on the closed lid for several minutes each day.

Where blepharitis is associated with sebor-rhoeic dermatitis or dandruff, treatment of the skin conditions may be undertaken at the same time as local treatment of the eyelids.

Where a blockage of the nasolacrimal duct is sus-pected (as with excessive lacrimation), an attempt can be made to resolve the problem by applying pressure with one finger to the lacrimal sac at the internal corner of the eye and lightly massaging the duct beneath. Failure to release fluid should not be followed by increasing the pressure. If the condition is troublesome, especially in children, an appointment should be made to see the doctor.

Patients should be reminded to take common-sense measures to reduce the irritant effects of environmental substances, such as dust, cosmet-ics, smoke and chlorine in swimming pools, where this is appropriate.

SUMMARY OF EYE DISORDERS

Blepharitis

Blepharitis is an inflammation of the glands of the margin of the eyelid, most noticeably the eyelash roots. It may be allergic in origin and a long-standing allergic reaction can often produce blepharoconjunctivitis, which is treated in the same way as allergic conjunctivitis. Blepharitis is also sometimes caused by infection. It can also be associated with seborrhoea of the scalp or face.

Cataract

A cataract is an opacity of the lens, most commonly seen in the elderly as a result of degenerative changes with age (Figure 5.9). It presents with some kind of visual impairment and usually occurs in both eyes. Surgery is the treatment of choice – **refer**.

Conjunctivitis

Conjunctivitis is an inflammation of the conjunctiva (the membrane covering the eye, except for the cornea, and the inner surface of the eyelids). It may be allergic in origin or infective, the most common bacterial cause being *Staphylococcus aureus*. The conjunctiva are inflamed, red and oedematous (see Figure 5.3) and the patient complains of itchiness or grittiness on the surface of the eye. In infective conjunctivitis, there is usually a discharge, which may be purulent.

Corneal ulcer

Ulceration of the cornea may be caused by infection or injury and is characterised by pain (though this is not invariably present), photophobia and either dryness or lacrimation. In severe cases there may be visual impairment. The ulcers may be visible, particularly if illuminated from an oblique side angle, when the catchlight reflects their shape – **refer**.

Dacrocystitis

Dacrocystitis is an inflammation of the lacrimal sac, which drains tears into the nasolacrimal duct from which they are drained into the nasal cavity. An obstruction of the nasolacrimal duct or, in children, a failure of the duct to open, also results in dacrocystitis – **refer** if gentle massage of the corner of the eye does not relieve obstruction.

→

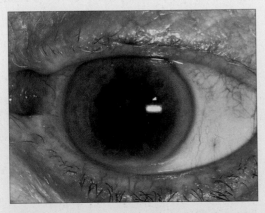

Figure 5.9   Cataract. (Reproduced with permission from Dr P. Marazzi/Science Photo Library.)

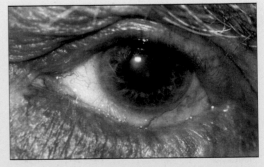

Figure 5.10   Entropion: the lower eyelid is inverted. (Reproduced with permission from the Science Photo Library.)

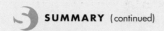 **SUMMARY** (continued)

Dry eye
Dry eye is a chronic disorder often associated with some underlying systemic disease. The conjunctiva, sclera and cornea can be affected, causing superficial irritation and sometimes photophobia. If untreated it may lead to corneal ulceration – **refer**.

Ectropion and entropion
Occasionally, and usually in the elderly, the eyelids may become displaced. They may invert (entropion; Figure 5.10) so that the lid margins and eyelashes abrade and irritate the surface of the eye, or evert (ectropion; Figure 5.11), so that the lids, particularly the lower one, fall away from the eye, offering it insufficient protection and lubrication. In both conditions there is an overflow of tears. In ectropion the lower lid may become chronically infected and scarred. In entropion, the lashes may fall out and infection may follow. As with ectropion, if seen relatively early on, a minor surgical procedure can correct the displacement. If left untreated it may lead to corneal ulceration because of trauma from the inverted lashes and poor lubrication of the tissues.

Glaucoma
Glaucoma is characterised by an increase in the intraocular pressure, caused by an imbalance between production and drainage of the aqueous humour (Figure 5.12). Closed-angle (narrow-angle) glaucoma is caused by obstruction to the drainage of the aqueous humour, often due to the position and shape of the iris. The condition produces severe pain within the eye and often headache, nausea and vomiting. Acute glaucoma generally affects one eye only. The visual field may be affected, often at night when haloes will be seen around lights. Open-angle (chronic simple) glaucoma develops gradually over a number of years, usually affecting both eyes. Symptoms occur insidiously and may present as headaches and loss in the visual field. By the time that symptoms are obvious, irreversible retinal damage will have occurred. Every adult consulting the pharmacist with an eye disorder represents an opportunity to reinforce the need for regular checks by an optometrist who will measure the intraocular pressure and is thus able to make the diagnosis in its early stages. Both types of glaucoma will lead to blindness if untreated – **refer**.

(continued overleaf)

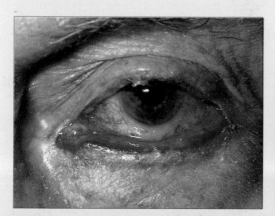

Figure 5.11 Ectropion of the lower eyelid, where the eyelid falls away from the eye. (Reproduced with permission from Dr P. Marazzi/Science Photo Library.)

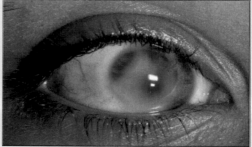

Figure 5.12 Late changes seen in glaucoma, showing clouding of the iris. (Reproduced with permission from Dr P. Marazzi/Science Photo Library.)

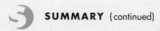 **SUMMARY** (continued)

Iritis (uveitis)

Iritis is an inflammation of the iris. Associated structures, such as the ciliary body (iridocyclitis), are often involved. The condition may be caused by infection or allergy or may be the result of systemic disease. Symptoms include pain within the eye, photophobia, visual impairment and hazy, small, irregularly shaped and unreactive pupils. Iritis may progress to cause cataracts (if the lens is involved) or glaucoma (if the angle at the edge of the ciliary body is eliminated). There is a danger of permanent visual loss unless diagnosis and treatment occurs at an early stage. It is often recurrent – **refer**.

Meibomian cyst (chalazion)

A meibomian cyst may be described as an internal stye or abscess affecting the meibomian glands situated deep in the cartilaginous tissue of the eyelids. It appears as a hard red lump which may be seen and felt under either the upper or lower lid (see Figure 5.7), but it is generally painless. The condition will resolve itself and is not serious. However, if it recurs frequently, referral is advised to treat any locus of infection.

Ptosis

Ptosis is drooping of the upper eyelid (see Figure 5.8). It can be caused by impairment of the musculature or by systemic disease – **refer**.

Styes

A stye is a staphylococcal infection of a hair follicle gland at the base of an eyelash, causing redness and irritation and possibly progressing to pain and swelling of the eyelid (see Figure 5.5). Styes are common and often recurrent.

Subconjunctival haemorrhage

With subconjunctival haemorrhage, a part of the conjunctiva covering the white of the eye appears bright red as a result of a haemorrhage in a small vessel (see Figure 5.4). It is harmless and resolves spontaneously after several weeks – **refer** if recurrent.

WHEN TO REFER
Eye disorders

- Pain within the eye (in contrast to superficial itchiness, grittiness or soreness)
- Disturbance in vision
- Pupils appear abnormal or uneven
- Pupils have abnormal or uneven reaction to light
- Upper eyelid drooping (ptosis)
- Recurrent lump under upper eyelid
- Recurrent subconjunctival haemorrhage
- Babies under three months old
- Babies with a squint
- Existing eye disease
- Bulging of eyes (proptosis)
- Dry eyes (unless previously seen by the doctor)

Accompanying symptoms
- Headache

CASE STUDIES

Case 1

A man in his mid 60s approaches the pharmacist with a prescription for an ophthalmic topical beta-blocker, something he has never had before. The pharmacist checks he is familiar with its use.
'You don't remember me, do you?' he enquires.

It transpires he visited several months ago with a simple conjunctivitis, probably allergic. The advice he received then included having a routine eye test, long overdue. This he did, although the importance of it escaped him at the time, until a raised intraocular pressure was discovered and this prescription was the eventual outcome.

'I don't know whether to thank you or not', he concludes. 'I'm told I shall be using these drops for the rest of my life.'

'Surely better than risking blindness,' argues the pharmacist.

'But my vision is perfect!' he exclaims, adding that he had a friend with glaucoma who had suffered sudden, terrible pain in one eye and immediate deterioration of his eyesight. No one would ignore that.

Smiling, the pharmacist explains that the patient's friend almost certainly had acute glaucoma – different cause, very serious, and although much rarer, certainly unmistakable. This man's problem, however, is chronic glaucoma: insidious onset, with no symptoms and the visual loss only evident when it becomes advanced and permanent. It is possibly the most important reason for having regular checks.

The gentleman looks thoughtful for a moment, and then returns the smile.

'I'd better get home,' he says. 'I cancelled the wife's appointment. Said we couldn't afford it!'

(continued overleaf)

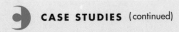

CASE STUDIES (continued)

Case 2

A young man, a university student, seeks advice. The problem is watery eyes – hay fever he believes, as several of his friends suffer from it. However, he has no rhinitis or other symptoms, he just has a sudden highly irritating conjunctivitis, with profuse lacrimation, which he finds debilitating and often socially embarrassing.

On enquiry this condition has no obvious relationship to the weather, pollen count or the season of the year. The pharmacist seeks other possible contact irritants, but can find none. About to give up, the student admits that there is one possibility: eating certain kinds of fruit seems to trigger it. He knows of the association with strawberries and some shellfish, but in his case it is apples. He has not mentioned it before, believing he might be ridiculed.

On the contrary, says the pharmacist, it is more common than usually thought. It is possible to have skin tests to learn more, but this is probably unnecessary when the cause is obvious. The pharmacist recommends eye-drops containing an antihistamine combined with a sympathomimetic agent to keep with him and use at the onset. This should alleviate the conjunctivitis in 15 to 30 minutes.

The young man leaves, with profound thanks. Whether these are for the medication or for taking the apple theory seriously, the pharmacist will never be sure.

Case 3

An elderly gentleman is very concerned. He has had a haemorrhage. The truth behind this alarming statement is a subconjunctival haemorrhage, but he believes this is indicative of deeper, perhaps cerebral, pathology.

The pharmacist is able to reassure him that this is not the case, and that the bleeding is tiny and from a capillary within the sclera. Even so, it looks spectacular, and as it resolves through the usual colours of a bruise, it may take a week, maybe two, to resolve.

It is considered good practice, however, to check the blood pressure of any patient with a subconjunctival haemorrhage, and the pharmacist advises the man to consult a nurse at the practice. The pharmacist also notes from the medication record that this man is taking warfarin, and advises that the INR too should be checked, adding that in the pharmacist's experience both are usually completely normal. They were duly checked, and were indeed normal. But the pharmacist was wrong about the haemorrhage: it took three weeks to resolve.

6

Constipation

The normal bowel habit can vary between individuals from twice daily to once every two or three days. Constipation may therefore mean different things to different people. It is important to ask a patient what they mean when they complain of constipation to ensure that the problem is real and not imagined. Generally, the following two criteria should be fulfilled: firstly, there is a change in bowel frequency from the norm for that patient and, secondly, hard stools are passed, often with difficulty and straining.

The causes of constipation range from simple changes in lifestyle and daily routine to major bowel or systemic disease.

Assessing symptoms

Duration

Simple transient constipation will resolve spontaneously within a few days. As a general rule of thumb, it is not necessary to treat acute constipation until the symptom has been present for four days, provided that no other symptoms are present. The actual time-scale will obviously depend on the previous frequency of bowel movement in individual patients. If constipation has persisted for up to 14 days then an OTC laxative should be tried for four days. Should there be no bowel movement within this period, a referral is recommended.

In some patients, particularly young children and the elderly, constipation may arise from a failure to respond to the desire to defaecate. Over a period of months or years this may lead to chronic habitual constipation. If untreated, this may lead to stasis and loss of tone in the muscle of the colon, which in turn may progress to megacolon (permanent dilatation of the large bowel), thus making peristalsis difficult without resort to stimulant laxatives. Bowel habit may be less than once weekly.

Onset

Possible causes of constipation may be elicited by asking about recent events and changes in lifestyle that may have coincided with the onset of symptoms. For example, changes in the diet, such as reduced fibre intake (particularly fruit and vegetables) or a reduced overall intake (as in dieting or illness), will change the frequency of defaecation.

Dehydration caused either by a reduced fluid intake or by prescribing of diuretics will lower the water content of the large bowel and result in hard faeces, which may be difficult to pass. Elderly patients with a low fluid intake are particularly susceptible.

Changes in lifestyle, such as a change in job, shift work, a change in eating places or a lack of exercise (in bedridden patients or those on holiday from an active job), can all contribute to a reduced bowel frequency.

Concurrent disease (see below) and certain drugs (see Table 6.1) may be the cause of constipation in some cases. Also, various physiological changes to the body, as occur in old age and in pregnancy, cause constipation.

Table 6.1 Drugs causing constipation

Aluminium (e.g. antacids)
Anticholinergics
Antidiarrhoeal drugs (imprudent use)
Antihistamines (instrinsic anticholinergic activity)
Antitussives (e.g. codeine, pholcodine)
Diuretics (if dehydration occurs)
Iron
L-dopa
Opioid analgesics
Phenothiazines (intrinsic anticholinergic acitivity)
Tricyclic antidepressants (intrinsic anticholinergic acitivity)
Verapamil

Accompanying symptoms

General malaise

If the patient feels ill or unable to work while having constipation this should be regarded as unusual and a referral to the doctor made to exclude any underlying organic cause. The same applies to any fever or night sweats that the patient may mention.

Blood in the stool

Blood noticed on defaecation will have a perfectly innocent explanation in the vast majority of cases. Blood noticed as specks or as a light smear on the toilet paper after a bowel movement is most likely to be due to haemorrhoids or a fissure in the anal canal or the skin surrounding it. Straining at stool can cause or exacerbate haemorrhoids. Fresh blood present only on the surface of the stool has most likely come from the anus or the most distal part of the colon. Blood that is mixed with the faeces giving a dark colour, often described as tarry, may have a more serious cause, such as diverticulosis, a bleeding peptic ulcer or, rarely, a carcinoma.

Patients taking iron tablets often have a darkened stool, which is of no consequence.

Unless a previous diagnosis of haemorrhoids or a similar condition has been made by a doctor, and there has been no change in the severity of bleeding, it is wise to recommend all patients with rectal bleeding to visit their doctor for assessment of the cause. If small amounts of blood are seen, as described above, which fit a known diagnosis, then the constipation may be treated by the pharmacist in the normal way for a few days.

Pain

Continuous or severe abdominal pain accompanying constipation, which has been present for two days or more, requires a medical opinion. In particular, the pharmacist should be alert to the possibility of obstruction in the bowel (possibly caused by a tumour). In such cases, colicky pain, abdominal distension and vomiting may be present in addition to constipation that is total, i.e. neither stool nor air is passed.

Nausea or vomiting

The presence of nausea or vomiting with constipation should be regarded as an unusual sign and referral for a medical opinion should be made to exclude the possibility of an obstruction.

Weight loss

In common with many other disease areas, sudden weight loss for no obvious reason is a suspicious sign that requires referral for the doctor to exclude malignancy.

Diarrhoea

In young adults, alternating bouts of diarrhoea and constipation, together with abdominal pain, are typical of the irritable bowel syndrome. In elderly patients, such symptoms are suggestive of spurious (overflow) diarrhoea. If irritable bowel syndrome has been previously diagnosed by the doctor, bulk-forming laxatives are useful when constipation is the predominate symptom. Failure to control symptoms in this way requires referral. Suspicion of spurious diarrhoea in the elderly requires investigation and treatment by the doctor.

Concurrent disease

Hypothyroidism can manifest itself as constipation, together with lethargy and slowness of movement and mental activity. Depression has been said to cause constipation, although this may be related to treatment with tricyclic antidepressants in some cases (see Table 6.1).

Patients who have angina or have recently suffered a myocardial infarction may require laxatives if straining at stool causes chest pain.

Recurrence

Constipation that recurs without obvious cause or with increasing frequency, in the absence of any association with prescribed drugs, may reflect some underlying pathological cause, which should be investigated by a doctor.

Special considerations

Pregnancy

During the second and third trimesters of pregnancy an increased amount of circulating progesterone causes relaxation of the smooth muscle of the bowel. This, together with physical compression of the bowel by the growing uterus and the effects of iron therapy, often results in constipation. Other changes in lifestyle in pregnancy, such as reduced exercise and eating fads, increase the tendency to develop constipation. Patients can be reassured that the symptom is a natural response of the bowel to pregnancy. Treatment is necessary with OTC laxatives, such as bulking agents or senna, if dietary management is not successful because haemorrhoids may develop if constipation is allowed to persist in pregnancy.

Age

Babies who are being breast fed normally produce fewer stools than bottle-fed babies. This is perfectly normal and does not require any intervention. Constipation in a bottle-fed baby may be caused by insufficient water being added to the milk powder. Babies, or older children, who become irritable, feverish or drowsy or who scream, have pain, feed or eat less or vomit should be referred.

Older children may develop phobias about toileting or may refuse to respond to the call to stool in order to attract attention. This has the desired effect of producing anxiety in the parent, who may become obsessive about regularising the bowel habit of the child.

Constipation that is more than transient should be viewed with more suspicion the older the patient is, since bowel cancer becomes increasingly more common above the age of about 50 years.

With increasing age, muscle tone in the bowel is reduced and faecal stasis can occur. In elderly patients regularity of the bowel habit can be an obsession and they will use laxatives not only to restore the habit to normal but also as a prophylaxis against any future possibility of constipation. This can lead to chronic laxative abuse, causing more reduction in bowel muscle tone and chronic constipation.

Constipation in the elderly should be taken seriously as it may reflect a state of dehydration that requires rectifying. A bowel filled with impacted faeces may compress adjacent structures such as the urinary tract and cause urinary retention.

Some elderly patients with impacted faeces may have concomitant diarrhoea. This is caused by small amounts of liquid stool being forced past the impacted stool in the rectum, causing a so-called spurious or overflow diarrhoea.

Management

For patients who have constipation of short duration (less than 14 days), the short-term relief of symptoms should be obtained by a laxative. Stimulant laxatives provide the most rapid effect, while osmotic laxatives and bulking agents usually have an onset of action of two to three days.

The cornerstone of long-term management is dietary advice, emphasising the value of fibre and fluid intake. Second-line treatment is the use of bulk laxatives.

Indiscretions in the diet, particularly a lack of fruit and vegetables or an inadequate fluid intake, are often responsible for bouts of constipation. Reduced intake of refined carbohydrate, such as sugar, cakes and pastry, and education regarding a healthy diet and exercise will often solve the problem without resort to using laxatives.

As already stated, with the standard western diet some people will have a bowel movement only once every two to three days. There is, however, evidence that such patterns are associated with an increased incidence of bowel problems, such as diverticular disease, and even more sinister problems, including cancer. There is a school of thought that everyone should have a bowel movement at least once per day and that the diet should be changed or at least extra fibre added until this occurs.

Laxatives may be divided into four categories: bulk, stimulant, osmotic and stool softeners. Liquid paraffin, a lubricant laxative, was popular in the past, but its use is now deprecated because of its many potential adverse effects. These include seepage from the oesophagus into the airways and lungs with devastating effects, and a tendency to reduce the absorption of fat-soluble vitamins.

Bulk-forming laxatives

Bulking agents act by retaining water in the large bowel, thus increasing stool bulk and stimulating bowel movement, resulting in a soft stool. They usually take several days to exert a significant effect. Examples include methylcellulose, sterculia, ispaghula husk and bran.

They are relatively safe to use and are popular because they are inert substances which mimic the natural action of fibrous food in the bowel. They can be recommended to both young and elderly patients and are safe for use in pregnancy.

Bulk-forming laxatives should be taken with plenty of fluid to speed transit along the alimentary tract, since cases of oesophageal and bowel obstruction have been reported. This is particularly important in elderly patients, who may have a reduced fluid intake or difficulty in swallowing. Patients who take these agents with inadequate amounts of water immediately before retiring to bed will be prone to oesophageal obstruction.

Stimulant laxatives

Where bulking agents are inappropriate or ineffective, the stimulant laxatives (irritant or contact laxatives) may be considered, particularly for short-term or infrequent use. They are believed to stimulate nerve endings in the nerve plexuses of the bowel wall, causing increased peristalsis. They are quicker acting than the bulk laxatives and a bowel movement can be expected within eight to 12 hours of taking them. Examples include senna and bisacodyl. Both of these drugs are safe and effective. Traditional agents in this category of laxatives, such as castor oil, which is hydrolysed in the bowel to form ricinoleic acid, and phenolphthalein, should not be recommended because of the possibility of unpleasant adverse effects.

Senna is safe to use in pregnancy after the first trimester.

Bisacodyl suppositories (adult and paediatric dosage forms) can produce a bowel movement within one or two hours of insertion and are therefore useful when the patient wants a rapid result.

The chronic use of stimulant laxatives is associated with tolerance and bowel atony.

Patients with irritable bowel disease and diverticulosis may take these drugs in combination with bulk laxatives under medical advice.

Osmotic laxatives

Like bulking agents, osmotic laxatives retain fluid within the bowel to stimulate peristalsis and formation of a soft stool. They tend to be more powerful than the bulk-forming laxatives. The most common agents in this category are magnesium salts, such as magnesium sulphate (Epsom salts), and lactulose.

Magnesium sulphate has a rapid effect, while the onset of action of lactulose is generally two or three days. Magnesium salts are absorbed to some extent and chronic use is not recommended. They are best avoided, except as a single treatment, in patients with chronic renal disease.

Glycerin suppositories are believed to act by both a local osmotic action and a local stimulant effect. They can be confidently recommended for children and should produce a bowel action in one or two hours.

Stool softeners

The term 'stool softener' generally refers to those agents that act like detergents by reducing the surface tension of hard faeces in the bowel, allowing water to penetrate the faeces. The only drug in this category in common use is docusate sodium. It is useful in patients with haemor-rhoids who are constipated and may be valuable in the elderly or for constipation induced by codeine or prescribed opioids. In opioid-induced constipation it should be combined with a stimulant laxative, such as senna, to promote peristalsis.

Duration of treatment

As for the vast majority of conditions and symptoms treated with OTC medicines, a failure to produce relief in seven to 14 days should alert the pharmacist to recommend that the patient seeks a medical opinion. This is not only to exclude any significant cause of the constipation but also to prevent chronic use, leading to abuse of laxatives, particularly the stimulant type.

 SUMMARY OF CONDITIONS PRODUCING CONSTIPATION

Acute constipation
This is a change in bowel frequency from normal of a few days' duration. It results in the passage of hard stools. It is a common disorder and usually will respond to OTC laxatives within a few days.

Bowel obstruction
A mechanical or paralytic obstruction of the small or large bowel prevents passage of the stool. Causes include carcinoma, strictures, adhesions after surgery, strangulated bowel, hernias and inflammation. Symptoms include colicky pain, nausea or vomiting, constipation (of both flatus and stool) and eventually abdominal distension and shock – **refer**.

Carcinoma of the large bowel
Malignancy in the colon or rectum is more common in the middle aged and elderly and may be advanced before symptoms are either noticed or acted upon. Weight loss is common, often with general malaise, constipation, nausea or vomiting and appetite loss, and other symptoms described above under bowel obstruction. Blood in the stool (melaena) is a cardinal sign of a colonic or rectal tumour – **refer**.

Chronic habitual constipation
Constipation may arise from a low-fibre diet or failure to respond to the desire to pass a motion, and leads to chronic habitual constipation after several months. There may be a consequent loss of tone in the smooth muscle of the colon, leading to reduced peristalsis and constipation.

(continued overleaf)

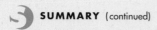

SUMMARY (continued)

Diverticular disease

Diverticulosis is a condition in which small pouches, called diverticuloae, appear in the mucosa of the large bowel and protrude down into the smooth muscle in the bowel wall. It is sometimes associated with a low-fibre diet. The disease is usually asymptomatic except when the diverticulae become inflamed or infected. The condition is then referred to as diverticulitis. There may be colicky abdominal pain, which is often left sided, caused by colonic spasm. Constipation and diarrhoea often alternate, sometimes with melaena. Treatment is with analgesics, spasmolytic drugs (such as hyoscine) and, where there is constipation, bulk laxatives along with a high-fibre diet. If a patient presents with an acute exacerbation of the condition or the condition has not been diagnosed – **refer.**

Haemorrhoids

Haemorrhoids are dilatations of veins engorged with blood, present either above (internal piles) or below (external piles) the anal sphincter. Pain is a common symptom, particularly after a bowel movement. Patients may suppress the call to stool in an attempt to avoid symptoms and this can result in constipation. The eventual passage of hard faeces irritates the haemorrhoids and thus a vicious circle may develop. If suspected but not previously diagnosed by a doctor – **refer.**

Irritable bowel syndrome

Irritable bowel syndrome (spastic colon) is characterised by abdominal colicky pain and a change in bowel habit which may be constipation or diarrhoea or alternate between both. On investigation, there is no detectable pathology or evidence of organic disease. The condition is common in young adults and emotion and stress are aggravating factors. Treatment should be tailored to individual symptoms with spasmolytics, analgesics, high-fibre diet and bulk-forming laxatives (see also Chapter 7).

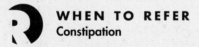

WHEN TO REFER
Constipation

- Abdominal pain
- Duration longer than 14 days without improvement, particularly in the elderly and patients with diabetes, hypothyroidism, haemorrhoids or Parkinson's disease, and those who have had strokes or are aged over 40 who present with a sudden change in bowel habit for the first time
- Patients taking long-term laxatives, unless prescribed by the doctor
- Children under one year old – advise discussion with the health visitor
- Constipation and not passing flatus
- Fluctuating constipation and diarrhoea, unless already investigated by the doctor

Accompanying symptoms
- Vomiting
- Rectal bleeding
- Thirst

CASE STUDIES

Case 1

A pleasant woman, well known to her pharmacist, calls in to collect the routine prescription for her elderly mother. The pharmacist remembers her mother, a thin frail woman with osteoporosis and a degree of cardiac failure, and asks after her.

The mother often collects her own prescription, but apparently recently has felt tired and listless, and has not been as active as formerly. The doctor saw her once, when she had a chest infection. That cleared up with treatment and the doctor could find nothing else of significance. She has also become constipated and the pharmacist and daughter agree that perhaps a laxative might help. The pharmacist is about to recommend a bulk-increasing agent but, on checking her medication record notices she is taking what appears to be large quantities of diuretics. The daughter agrees. The dosage was increased some time ago, when her mother developed oedema, and as so often happens it has remained high ever since. She is often thirsty (diabetes having been excluded), has possibly lost a little weight, although she is underweight anyway, and eats poorly. She has also become incontinent of urine at times, which has been attributed to her diuretics but probably is in part due to the constipation.

The pharmacist can see no harm in short-term relief of her symptoms with appropriate treatment, but strongly recommends she makes an appointment with the doctor for a review of her medication.

Constipation in the elderly is often regarded as inevitable, but treatable causes can be found in some people, and medication is one of the more common causes.

Case 2

A middle-aged woman is a frequent visitor to both her doctor and the pharmacy. She often states that her irritable bowel controls her life. She juggles with a variety of treatments, some of which work for some of the time.

Her bowels are among the things she attempts to regulate. On this occasion diarrhoea is the problem. She has colicky abdominal pains, flatulence and frequent semi-liquid stools. She usually takes codeine phosphate to alleviate these symptoms, and presents a prescription from her long list of repeat medications.

A few days later she returns. The pain is worse, rather than better, and she would like to buy a paracetamol–codeine combination to deal with it. She emphasises that she understands the pharmacist's reluctance to recommend the two products together, but maintains that she has studied the condition for years and knows her own body better than anyone. Even so, argues the pharmacist, two products containing codeine cannot be recommended and therefore the pharmacist feels unable to comply, at least without a further prescription from the doctor. The pharmacist also feels slightly guilty at passing the buck to the doctor. As an attempt to pacify the situation, the pharmacist enquires a little further – there is rarely any problem in persuading this woman to discuss her symptoms. The pain is, she alleges, slightly relieved with a bowel action; she has low abdominal discomfort and a sense of fullness with incomplete emptying. The pharmacist wonders if this is simply diarrhoea or if it represents constipation with overflow. If it were the latter her self-medication will only aggravate it. She dismisses the theory, suggesting that it has been invented to suit the pharmacist's end. She leaves for the doctor's surgery.

When the woman returns, it is with a prescription for an osmotic laxative. With care, the prescription is accepted, dispensed and handed out with no eye contact or word spoken between them.

(continued overleaf)

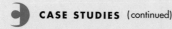

Case 3

A rather nervous young man whispers to the pharmacist, 'piles'. He is taken to one side, and further enquiries made. Gradually, and with some embarrassment, the pharmacist learns of a history of only a few weeks, pain and occasionally a tender lump present, with bleeding on one occasion only – just a smear on the paper.

The diagnosis is obvious; the patient is in his mid 20s, so the risk of malignancy is negligible, and a suitable topical product is advised. The consultation has not been easy, and both parties are pleased to see it over.

However, two weeks later the man returns with the same secretive story. The cream has failed. 'Suppositories?' wonders the pharmacist, although the required explanation seems daunting, and so the pharmacist questions a little more. The patient has recently left the family home, where the food was wholesome and regular. Now working long hours for a computer company he eats in the canteen, where the menu is fast, prepared well in advance and very different to what he is used to. The result: constipation. The pharmacist explains the connection between his new life style and his distressing complaint, although when describing the hazards of straining at stool it is obvious the young man is no longer listening.

Time, however, proves the pharmacist's words not to have been wasted. The young man's mother was equally distraught at this development in his career, and he now sports a lunch box full of whole-wheat sandwiches and fresh fruit. What he told his mother to acquire these feasts remains a mystery.

7

Diarrhoea

Diarrhoea is a symptom requiring a clear quantitative description by the sufferer, since its definition will vary considerably between patients. A general definition would be a change in normal bowel habit resulting in increased frequency of bowel movements and the passage of soft or watery motions. It is often accompanied by colicky pain. Thus, at one end of the spectrum, diarrhoea may present as frequent, formed, small stools and at the other as frequent, voluminous, watery motions. The difference may sometimes be useful in assessing the severity of a patient's condition.

The commonest type of diarrhoea presenting in the pharmacy is acute diarrhoea and the most likely causes are dietary insults or bacterial or viral infection. The vast majority of these cases will resolve spontaneously in two or three days without any specific treatment.

Chronic diarrhoea that lasts for weeks rather than days may indicate a pathological cause. It may represent the recurrence or flare up of a previously diagnosed disorder, such as irritable bowel syndrome, or a problem that requires medical referral for investigation and diagnosis.

Assessing symptoms

Severity and type

The severity of diarrhoea may be arbitrarily graded in terms of frequency, volume, duration and the presence of particular accompanying symptoms.

Any patient who suffers severe malaise or pain with diarrhoea for more than one or two days, without any sign of improvement, should be referred.

Duration

The common acute types of diarrhoea caused by viruses or bacteria (the latter usually from contaminated food or water) generally resolve spontaneously in two to three days. It is therefore reasonable to wait to see if improvement occurs before making any decision to refer, unless concomitant symptoms dictate otherwise.

Persistent night-time diarrhoea requires medical appraisal for the presence of inflammatory bowel disease, such as Crohn's disease or ulcerative colitis.

In young children with diarrhoea, the timescale for referral should be shorter than for older children or adults (see Special considerations).

Chronic diarrhoea, i.e. lasting for several days, weeks or longer, or recurrent episodes of diarrhoea usually indicate major pathology, requiring referral. However, in many instances the patient will have a known diagnosis, such as irritable bowel syndrome, inflammatory bowel disease, diverticular disease or some malabsorption syndrome, and they will have been advised how to treat the symptoms by their doctor.

Onset

The patient should be questioned to establish if the onset of symptoms was associated with any particular event. Symptoms occurring within 72 hours of eating food, particularly dairy products, poultry or meat, especially if others who ate the same food have the same symptoms, suggest a bacterial cause. Onset within six hours of eating those foods, together with vomiting, and again,

Table 7.1 Drugs that may cause diarrhoea
Antibiotics
Colchicine
Iron
Laxatives (overuse or abuse)
Magnesium antacids
Metformin
NSAIDs, especially mefenamic acid and indometacin

if the symptoms are shared with others who ate the same food, suggests infection with pre-formed toxins from bacteria.

Association with drug therapy (see Table 7.1) or particular foods should be inquired about. It may be possible to identify an intolerance or allergy to particular food items, such as mushrooms, milk or alcohol (usually beer in large amounts).

Recent travel to tropical or subtropical countries may indicate diarrhoea related to contamination of food or water (so called travellers' diarrhoea). This is usually of short duration. Persistent symptoms might signify more serious infection, such as bacterial or protozoal dysentery, cholera (bacterial) or giardiasis (protozoal).

Accompanying symptoms

Concurrent disease

In addition to previously diagnosed disorders of the bowel, other conditions may cause secondary diarrhoea. For example, hyperthyroidism and diabetes can cause diarrhoea, the latter as a result of either disease of the autonomic nerves in the bowel in long-standing and poorly controlled diabetes or the effect of drug treatment.

Abdominal pain

Abdominal discomfort is common in patients with diarrhoea. It may present as a sharp, colicky or griping pain, usually in the central region of the abdomen, and it is generally of no signifi-

cance. However, severe abdominal pain, which is not resolving, requires referral.

Rarely, abdominal pain with diarrhoea may represent irritation of the bowel by an inflamed appendix. In such cases the stools are usually not watery or profuse but merely unformed. Acute appendicitis usually begins with pain in the central abdominal region or right flank and there is right-sided tenderness. The pain is continuous, except when perforation occurs, when the pain suddenly stops for one or two hours and then starts again. The pain of appendicitis wakes the patient at night.

Left-sided pain or tenderness, accompanied by either diarrhoea alone, or sometimes by alternating episodes of diarrhoea and constipation, may be a sign of diverticular disease.

Vomiting

Vomiting and diarrhoea suggest an infective gastroenteritis caused by a virus or bacteria, the latter often from a food source.

Weight loss

Significant weight loss over a few weeks may be a symptom of a previously diagnosed illness causing chronic diarrhoea. However, in all cases where a diagnosis has not previously been made, referral is necessary to exclude tumours (particularly in the elderly) or malabsorption syndromes.

Blood and mucus in stool

Blood in the stool is usually a signal to refer the patient, especially if it is persistent. Bloody diarrhoea occurs in inflammatory bowel disease (along with the passage of mucus or pus) and cancer of the colon.

Mucus in the stool is a sign of acute inflammation of the large bowel lining and may present either when there is serious pathology or when there is an acute episode of a less serious, self-remitting condition. It is thus not diagnostic nor worrying on its own, but should be considered as a sign for referral if it persists or if it is accompanied by other worrying symptoms such as blood in the stool.

Frequency and urgency of micturition

Frequency and urgency of urination are commonly present when there is diarrhoea, which is essentially frequency and urgency of defaecation. This is caused by the proximity of the colon and the urinary tract, and the general reflex irritability of smooth muscle in the walls of these hollow organs.

Dyspareunia (painful intercourse)

Dyspareunia in women is sometimes a symptom complained of by sufferers of irritable bowel syndrome. It may be due to proximity to an inflamed or distended colon, although it can be exacerbated by stress.

Upper respiratory symptoms

Symptoms of the common cold occurring at the same time as diarrhoea suggest a viral infection.

Fever

A fever, with or without malaise, suggests infection. This may be monitored for a few days in adults, unless the patient has recently returned from a tropical or subtropical country, in which case referral is necessary to exclude diagnoses such as dysentery and malaria.

Diarrhoea alternating with constipation

In young adults episodes of diarrhoea alternating with constipation may indicate irritable bowel syndrome. In this syndrome the complaint of constipation can occur when the stool is normal in form but after evacuation the patient feels that the stool is still there; this is known as 'rectal dissatisfaction'. In the elderly this may be a sign of spurious diarrhoea (see p 66). As irritable bowel syndrome is essentially a disorder of function, disturbing the normal motility of the large bowel, a common clinical pattern is one of increasingly difficult episodes of constipation eventually relieved by diarrhoea, although with stasis and distension and then overflow the pattern is often less obvious.

Other chronic symptoms

As mentioned above, patients with a diagnosed chronic condition will often suffer from other long-term symptoms apart from their chronic diarrhoea, and the majority of patients will be familiar with these and able to cope with them. Such symptoms may include abdominal pain, bloating and abdominal distension, nausea and fatigue. Unless there is a sudden change in the severity of these accompanying symptoms or an otherwise unexpected occurrence, reassurance and, if appropriate, simple symptomatic treatment are all that is required.

Aggravating factors

It is well known that stress or anxiety can induce or exacerbate diarrhoea. Although this is typical of the history of irritable bowel syndrome, which is seen particularly in young adults, it is not exclusive to this condition.

Apart from any causative agent involved, diarrhoea may be worsened by dietary changes such as an increase in fibre or fat content, spices, alcohol or even an excess of tea or coffee.

Incidence and recurrence

Continuous or recurrent diarrhoea strongly suggests some underlying cause and requires a medical opinion.

Nocturnal diarrhoea, other than that experienced immediately after a digestive insult, should be regarded as unusual. Referral is needed to exclude diagnoses such as inflammatory bowel disease.

Diarrhoea caused by drugs will recur in association with administration of the offending agents. Patients should always be asked about current medication.

The presence of symptoms in other members of the household who share toilet facilities may indicate cross-infection or someone acting as a carrier, both of which can cause transference by the faecal–oral route.

Special considerations

Children

In babies the cause of diarrhoea may be infection and parents should be advised to take special care when sterilising bottles. Some cases of diarrhoea in bottle-fed babies will be caused by insufficient dilution of the milk, resulting in osmotic diarrhoea. Lactose intolerance can also lead to osmotic diarrhoea.

Very young children are at increased risk of dehydration. Babies under six months old with stools that are loose and more frequent than normal should be referred after 24 hours if the condition is not improving.

Children under two years old who have diarrhoea for more than 48 hours should be referred if they seem unwell or are not drinking normally.

Dehydration can be difficult to judge, but a limp, non-alert baby should be referred as soon as possible. The important fact to remember is that diarrhoea causes water and electrolyte loss, which must be checked, particularly in young children, by giving adequate fluids and, if possible, electrolyte mixtures. Traditionally, treatment of children has also involved restricting food until the diarrhoea improves, but a more modern approach is described below (see Management).

Elderly

Elderly patients, like children, are susceptible to the dehydrating effect of diarrhoea, especially those who are taking diuretics and those whose fluid and food intake is poor. It is wise to operate similar guidelines for referral to those described for children under two years.

Faecal impaction in the elderly can give rise to constipation and a so-called spurious or overflow diarrhoea. In this condition hard faeces obstruct most of the diameter of the bowel lumen. However, some fluid faeces can seep past the impacted mass, leading to a loose, unformed stool that is produced in relatively small amounts. It is most common in the immobile, frail elderly. Treating this condition as diarrhoea will only cause more constipa-

tion. The patient should instead be referred for a rectal examination and disimpaction of the faeces.

Management

By the time symptoms occur, the bowel mucosa will have already been damaged by bacteria or toxins. It then becomes inflamed and cannot function normally to absorb fluids and electrolytes. Instead it secretes fluids into the gut and although the inflammation will normally subside within a few days, extra fluids are often needed to counteract the fluid loss. The cornerstone of treatment of acute diarrhoea therefore is to maintain an adequate fluid balance. This is particularly important in young children and the elderly. If the patient complains of thirst, this need should be satisfied so that lost body water can be replaced. In adults, bland, sugarless drinks, such as water or tea, should be given.

Fasting is generally not necessary if the patient wants to eat. This is also true for babies and children. Patients will, however, often report that food, even small amounts, goes right through them. Some authorities argue that fasting deprives infecting bacteria of nutrients in the bowel and thus shortens the illness. More recently others have argued it makes no difference to the outcome. It is difficult to give definitive guidelines on this issue.

Breast-fed babies should continue to feed since there is no evidence that this is deleterious. Although there is no evidence to show that fasting in bottle-fed babies is of any benefit, it is traditional to stop milk feeding for 24 hours, during which time a proprietary oral rehydration solution should be given instead. The next day, the milk feed should be diluted to a quarter of the normal concentration with water, followed by a 50 per cent dilution the next day, three-quarter strength the next day and finally upgrading to full strength. Fluids or diluted milk feeds should be offered at least every three hours. This will maintain nutrition and fluids at the desired level.

Oral rehydration solutions

Oral rehydration solutions are particularly suitable for babies and children. The sachets of powder contain electrolytes and glucose. The powders require mixing with water according to the manufacturer's instructions to prevent overloading. A simple rule of thumb is to give one cupful of solution for every loose stool to babies under one year and two cupfuls for older children. As a general rule, over the course of one or two days, the passage of up to four loose motions per day will not put any child at risk of dehydration. However, if the child is particularly ill or there are abnormal signs, such as unsatisfied thirst, dry mouth, poor urine output, rapid breathing or drowsiness, referral is necessary.

Antidiarrhoeal drugs

Some authorities decry the use of antidiarrhoeals on the basis that they do not appear to shorten the duration of illness and any benefit is symptomatic. However, for social reasons patients will often insist that symptomatic treatment is desirable and antidiarrhoeal medicines have an obvious placebo effect.

Loperamide

OTC loperamide is an effective symptomatic treatment suitable for adults and children over 12 years old. It decreases bowel motility through its action on opioid receptors in the gut and does not possess the potential adverse effects of anticholinergic drugs such as belladonna dry extract, hyoscine and dicyclomine (dicycloverine). Like other antidiarrhoeal agents, it is not recommended for patients with inflammatory bowel disease except under medical supervision, since it may cause constipation, obstruction and dilation of the bowel (megacolon).

Mebeverine

Mebeverine is a directly acting spasmolytic drug that has no anticholinergic activity. It has been used for many years for the symptomatic treatment of irritable bowel syndrome and as such it appears to be effective in relieving the abdominal cramps and hypermotility of the large bowel with few adverse effects.

Alverine

Like mebeverine, alverine has no anticholinergic activity, but exerts a direct relaxant effect on the bowel smooth muscle and is also an acceptable treatment for the symptoms of irritable bowel syndrome.

Morphine

Traditional medicines, such as kaolin and morphine mixture, as well as a number of proprietary products containing morphine, are popular for the treatment of acute diarrhoea, although there is little objective evidence of their efficacy. However, they can lead to addiction if overused. Kaolin and morphine mixture has been reported to cause hypokalaemia because of the liquorice extract it contains, but this is unlikely unless there is chronic usage of large doses.

Codeine, an opioid-like morphine, is available in low dosage in some OTC products, but, like morphine, its efficacy at such doses is dubious and may be outweighed by its abuse potential.

Adsorbents

Adsorbents, such as kaolin, pectin and charcoal, have a traditional place in the mind of the public for the treatment of diarrhoea. They serve little useful therapeutic purpose although they may adsorb water in the bowel and add bulk to the stool. This may, however, lull patients into a false sense of security because they could still be losing large quantities of fluid from the bowel, but this will be less readily apparent because of the cosmetic effect of the adsorbent agent.

Bulk-forming agents

Bulking agents are usually used to treat constipation but they can be useful in conditions which produce chronic diarrhoea by absorbing water in the bowel and creating a formed stool. In irritable bowel syndrome, for instance, small doses of ispaghula or sterculia have been used to treat the diarrhoeal phase, but this should be tried carefully since the effect in some patients may be to worsen the flatus and bloating. There is some evidence that bran, in contrast to other types of fibre, may worsen the symptoms of irritable bowel syndrome, but this is controversial.

Peppermint oil

Formulations of peppermint oil have been designed to release the oil in the distal small bowel to avoid potential irritable effects in the mouth and oesphagus. Dispersion of the oil in the small bowel allows transport to the large bowel where the active ingredient, menthol, exerts a direct spasmolytic effect. It has been a popular prescribable treatment for irritable bowel syndrome for many years and is an acceptable addition to, or replacement for, other spasmolytic agents.

Advice for travellers abroad

The following pointers will help reduce the incidence of travellers' diarrhoea:

1. Drink bottled water or water sterilised with purification tablets
2. Avoid ice (unless personally made using bottled water) and ice cream
3. Avoid salads and uncooked vegetables (which may have been washed in contaminated water)
4. Avoid fruits that cannot be peeled
5. Avoid unpasteurised milk
6. Avoid murky swimming pools.

SUMMARY OF CONDITIONS PRODUCING DIARRHOEA

Carcinoma of the large bowel
A tumour in the large bowel can cause constipation or diarrhoea. Signs to look out for are blood in the stool, mucus in the stool (noticed as slime passed with the motion, often in the mornings), patient middle aged or older, abdominal pain, swelling in the abdomen and weight loss – **refer**. Any change in bowel habit in a patient aged over 50, particularly accompanied by weight loss or malaise, should be referred for investigation. Increasingly some surgeries and clinics are offering routine testing for occult blood and even sigmoidoscopy.

Diverticular disease
See Chapter 6, p 60.

Inflammatory bowel disease
Inflammatory bowel disease includes Crohn's disease, a disorder characterised by inflammation in any part of the digestive tract, including the large bowel, and ulcerative colitis, a disorder affecting the large bowel only. These conditions usually present in the teenage years and young adulthood. The classical symptoms are bloody diarrhoea, with repeated visits to the toilet that do not abate during the night. The

→

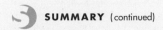

patient will feel ill and there will be weight loss and anorexia. The conditions are chronic, and are characterised by temporary remissions and flare ups – **refer**.

Food poisoning
Food poisoning is caused by bacteria such as *Salmonella, Campylobacter, Shigella, Clostridium* and *Staphylococcus.* Common sources of infection are meat, poultry and dairy products. In mild cases the condition is self-limiting over the course of one to three days. If symptoms (diarrhoea, vomiting and abdominal pain) are severe – **refer**.

Irritable bowel syndrome
Irritable bowel syndrome is a relatively common condition, affecting about 15 per cent of the population and often commencing in the under 40 age group. Symptoms vary among sufferers, but characteristically there is recurrent abdominal pain that is relieved by emptying the bowel, diarrhoea, which sometimes alternates with episodes of constipation, abdominal distension and bloating, a feeling of rectal fullness and incomplete evacuation. The diagnosis is often by exclusion of other conditions after the patient has had thorough tests and investigations. See also Chapter 6, p 60.

Malabsorption
Malabsorption syndromes, such as coeliac disease, are rare, but should be borne in mind when there is weight loss, fatigue or anaemia, with or without abdominal distension. In children, malabsorption is often associated with lactose intolerance.

Protozoal infection
Visitors to or from some tropical and subtropical countries may become infected with protozoa that cause diseases such as amoebic dysentery and giardiasis. These conditions may resolve spontaneously but if symptoms persist referral is advisable. Symptoms, in addition to diarrhoea, can include vomiting, abdominal pain, malaise and fever – **refer**.

Travellers' diarrhoea
Travellers' diarrhoea is an acute diarrhoea that may be caused by a change in diet (e.g. an increase in oily or spicy food), in climate or in the mineral content of drinking water. It is usually self-limiting but can be disruptive to holidays or business trips. If it persists, it may be due to infection, often with bacterial toxins such as from *Escherichia coli, Campylobacter* or *Shigella*. In some cases the infection may be viral. Infection usually occurs in a country where sanitary conditions are poor or drinking water is contaminated. Persistent cases require further investigation and referral.

Viral infections
Viral gastroenteritis is one of the most common types of diarrhoea in the UK in both children and adults. It is usually self-limiting.

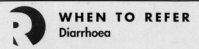

WHEN TO REFER
Diarrhoea

Onset
- Recent travel abroad   Medical opinion on the same day

Severity
- Patient obviously ill, e.g. showing signs   Refer urgently
  of dehydration, such as being delerious
  or confused, or small child with very
  dry mouth and lips

Duration
- Symptoms have changed or worsened
  and patient not improving after one or
  two weeks (depending on severity of
  original symptoms)

Accompanying symptoms
- Blood in stool   Same/next day
- Nausea (for more than three to four days)   Same/next day
- Loss of appetite (for more than three to four days)
- Weight loss (over previous two weeks)
- Fatigue
- Fever
- Pregnancy or breast feeding

Incidence
- Diarrhoea wakes patient at night several times for
  more than two or three consecutive nights

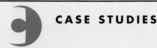

CASE STUDIES

Case 1

A well-dressed woman in her late 50s enters the pharmacy and requests a confidential word with the pharmacist. She and her husband have returned from a perfect Caribbean holiday, marred only on the last two days by intermittent abdominal pain and diarrhoea, which have persisted since their return. She is eager to point out that they stayed at a good hotel and were careful to observe the guide's recommendations. After noting the details, the pharmacist advises symptomatic relief in the short term, but stresses the need for further investigations, and points out that holiday diarrhoea, whatever its cause, does not reflect adversely on either the traveller or the resort.

A week later the woman returns, asking an assistant for more of the same medication. The pharmacist intervenes, repeating the advice given previously. The woman is now completely well but her husband, still unseen at the pharmacy, is worse, with more pain and diarrhoea that prevents him leaving the house. Away from the shop counter, she confidentially adds bleeding and the passage of mucus to the list of his symptoms. The pharmacist refuses to recommend further, and insists the woman calls the doctor, offering the use of the pharmacy telephone. The call is made and the woman returns home.

Another week passes before the woman returns, again requesting a quiet word. She asks for no sale, but wishes to thank the pharmacist, who saved her husband. Her husband is now in hospital, his diverticular abscess having been resected along with a length of colon shortly before it perforated, and is recovering. On leaving, a handsome donation finds its way into the charity box by the door.

Case 2

This young woman is well known to the pharmacy. She is smart and attractive in appearance, an air stewardess who from time to time purchases a variety of medicines, including analgesics and anti-inflammatories as well as her prescribed antispasmodics and oral contraceptives. She always listens intently to the advice offered, asking her own questions about drug safety and appropriateness.

One day she appears wanting 'a really strong laxative'. Recalling a prescription for a codeine containing analgesic only a couple of weeks before, the pharmacist feels this needs further exploration before a suitable recommendation is made. When told she may be taking medication that is aggravating her condition, she suddenly breaks down, her usual composure lost, and in tears is led to a quiet area along with a female assistant. The story is of several years of abdominal pain, bloating and varying bowel habit. She states it is ruining her life, her job and now threatening her relationship. Others have implied it is her lifestyle that has caused it. She has had seemingly endless tests, always humiliating yet always normal. She asks why the doctors cannot find out what is wrong and then treat it so she can get on with her life.

The pharmacist listens sympathetically and suggests starting at the beginning by sorting out her medication. After a telephone call to her doctor a few adjustments are made and follow-up arranged. Over the following weeks the pharmacist spends more time with the woman, monitoring her medication. With awkward working hours she is grateful to be able to call in when the opportunity arises, and during these calls the discussion broadens to her irregular hours and busy job, and a deep-seated feeling that she has no time to be ill.

Eventually she begins to accept the need to take some responsibility for her life, and for her irritable bowel syndrome, if she means to have any control over it. Her diet is discussed and she takes advice from the practice nurse. She stops smoking and becomes aware of her drinking pattern. She makes time

(continued overleaf)

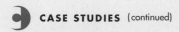

for regular exercise and for relaxation at the local health club. Gradually, through ups and downs, her symptoms improve and although to this day she still suffers relapses they are no longer the devastating intrusions they were.

Her boyfriend, however, did not see these benefits. She is now engaged, but to a man from outside the airline whose passion at weekends is cricket. His feet are firmly on the ground.

Case 3

A young woman, barely 20, comes to the pharmacy one Saturday afternoon. In a buggy she pushes her son, who is about one year old. She is anxious. The boy has had diarrhoea for three weeks. Everything he eats goes straight through him. She has been to the doctor repeatedly and the doctor has examined him, told her he is fine, and prescribed nothing. Now the surgery is closed, the weekend stretches before her and she feels she cannot cope. Her boyfriend and mother agree that something must be done.

The pharmacy is unexpectedly quiet, so the pharmacist takes a detailed history. The patient has never eaten well, always picks at food and is frequently at the doctor's with colds and coughs. This is the woman's first baby, and as she is receiving what feels like criticism from all sides she can only conclude that the problem must in some way be her fault.

Through all this, glances at the patient himself suggest a well-nourished, contented child. Slowly it emerges that the diarrhoea is in fact loose stools, but not invariably and not every day. Several times a week he produces voluminous and offensive motions, which spill from his nappy and soil both adjacent clothing and the atmosphere. Further questioning suggests an erratic diet. With a working mother, child-minders and grandparents, his diet is grazing, often unsuitable and mostly a selection of snacks rather than meals.

Reassurance is firm, with practical advice and positive reinforcement. The child is also teething, and this is addressed. An assistant with young children discusses nappies and children's diets. No medication is found necessary for the 'diarrhoea', but the mother leaves the shop considerably happier than when she came in and when, two weeks later, she returns to buy more nappies and teething gel, she does not make any reference to diarrhoea.

8

Abdominal disorders

One of the most common symptoms presented by patients to the pharmacist is abdominal discomfort or pain. This symptom encompasses a multitude of possible diagnoses relating to the gastrointestinal tract, the genito-urinary tract and sometimes other body systems from which pain may be referred to the abdomen.

A reasonably accurate diagnosis can often be made on the basis of a clear history, although sometimes the precise cause will remain a mystery. In such cases it is sufficient to determine the severity of the symptoms and the need for referral.

In this chapter, the term 'pain' is used to describe all symptoms ranging from a mild or vague discomfort, such as indigestion, to the more commonly accepted lay definition of pain as a sensation that hurts.

An important part of the history of a patient with abdominal symptoms is the location of the pain. The system used in medicine to describe the site of symptoms is to divide the abdomen into nine areas by mentally drawing across its surface two vertical and two horizontal lines, as shown in Figure 8.1.

Assessing symptoms

Location of pain

The information in Table 8.1 will be helpful in considering the possible cause of abdominal pain. It should be emphasised that this table indicates the sites where pain is typically felt, but there will be variability between individual patients and the presentation will not always be a classic textbook case. Abdominal pain is often not localised but will be described vaguely as covering all the abdomen. This may represent either a non-specific gastritis or enteritis with no known cause that will resolve spontaneously or, alternatively, the early presentation of a disorder that is not yet sufficiently advanced to show all of its typical features. Thus, the rest of the history must be considered along with questions about the site of pain.

Patients may give a clue to the diagnosis by the manner in which they show the location of their pain. In answer to the question 'Show me where the pain is', a patient with a peptic ulcer or other distinct lesion may point with a finger to an exact spot on the abdomen,

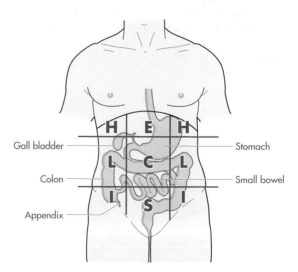

Figure 8.1 The nine areas of the abdomen used to locate symptoms (H, hypochondrium; E, epigastrium; L, loin; C, central; I, iliac fossa; S, suprapubic).

Table 8.1   Differential diagnosis of pain according to site

Chest
(Although anatomically distinct from the abdomen, symptoms felt in the chest may arise from the gastrointestinal tract)

Acid reflux, with or without hiatus hernia
Angina
Muscular strain
Myocardial infarction
Oesophagitis or oesophageal obstruction (difficulty in swallowing, lump in throat)
Peptic ulcer

Epigastric
Angina (atypical presentation)
Biliary colic (atypical presentation)
Gastritis/dyspepsia
Duodenitis
Oesophageal ulcer
Oesophageal reflux
Peptic ulcer (gastric or duodenal)
Pancreatitis
Tumour

Central
Abdominal aneurysm
Appendicitis (central pain which spreads after a few hours to the right iliac fossa)
Biliary colic (caused by infection of the gall bladder or common bile duct or obstruction with gallstone)
Bowel ischaemia
Colitis

Diverticular disease
Gastritis/gastroenteritis
Inflammatory bowel disease
Irritable bowel syndrome
Mesenteric adenitis
Obstruction
Pancreatitis
Peptic ulcer (gastric or duodenal)
Tumour

Suprapubic
Cystitis
Colitis
Diverticular disease
Irritable bowel syndrome
Tumour

Rectal pain
Rectal carcinoma
Haemorrhoids
Spasm of pelvic anal muscles

In women
Ovarian cyst
Salpingitis
Tubal (ectopic) pregnancy
Uterine disorders (e.g. dysmenorrhoea, endometriosis)

Hypochondrium
Either or both sides
Atypical presentation of pneumonia, pleurisy, angina
Muscular or ligamentous pain from the back
Peptic ulcer
Shingles

Left side
Gastritis

Right side
Biliary colic (often radiating to the back and shoulder)
Liver disease

Loin
Either or both sides
Lumbar muscle strain (felt in the lateral and posterior aspects of the loins)
Renal stone/ureteric colic
Shingles

Iliac Fossa
Either or both sides
Bowel tumour
Colitis
Diverticular disease

In women
Ovarian cyst
Salpingitis (inflammation of fallopian tubes)
Tubal (ectopic) pregnancy

Right side
Appendicitis

Groin Pain
Inguinal ligament strain (groin strain)
Inguinal or femoral hernia

Spread

whereas someone with a less specific symptom may place a whole hand over the area where the discomfort is felt. The typical locations of pain in common abdominal disorders are shown in Figure 8.2.

The pain of myocardial ischaemia, as in angina or infarction, is classically described as spreading from the chest to the jaw, neck, shoulder and arms. This helps to distinguish it from oesophagitis, although the classic radiation of

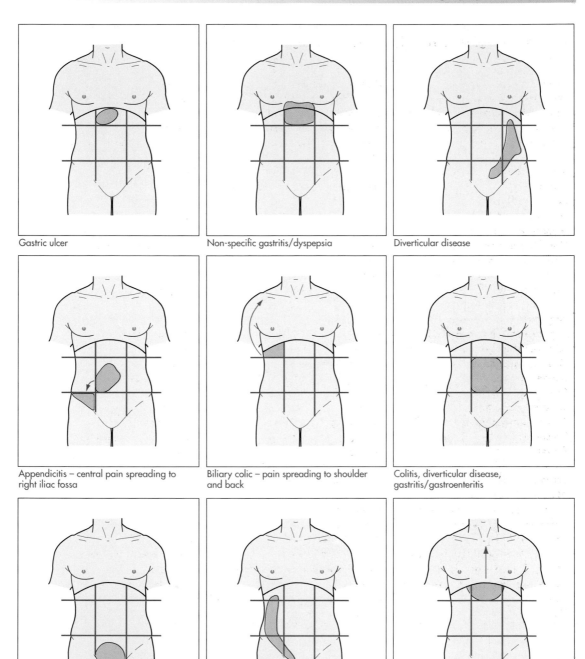

Gastric ulcer

Non-specific gastritis/dyspepsia

Diverticular disease

Appendicitis – central pain spreading to right iliac fossa

Biliary colic – pain spreading to shoulder and back

Colitis, diverticular disease, gastritis/gastroenteritis

Cystitis (infection in the bladder) – pain in the suprapubic area, often spreading to the back

Renal colic – left or right side, pain starts in the back and then spreads as stone moves down urinary tract

Oesophagitis, angina, myocardial infarction – in angina and myocardial infarction, pain can also spread to jaw, neck and arms

Figure 8.2 Typical location of pain in common abdominal disorders.

pain from the chest is not seen in every patient with cardiac ischaemia.

Appendicitis is often first felt as central pain, which radiates to the right iliac fossa after a few hours; again, this history will not be reported by every patient with appendicitis.

Pain that radiates to the back or shoulders is typical of biliary colic (e.g. due to gallstones), peptic ulcer and, more seriously, pancreatitis. The pain of cystitis may spread from the supra-pubic area to the back.

Pain in one loin that moves downwards into the suprapubic region or into the testis is typical of renal colic, caused by a stone passing from the kidney, along the ureter to the bladder and then the urethra. This journey of a stone may be spread over a long period of time (days or weeks).

Intensity and duration

Severe pain that is continuous for more than a few hours may indicate serious pathology and possibly a medical emergency. If there is no pre-vious history and the pain is sudden in onset, such severe pain is described clinically as an acute abdomen. It may be caused by conditions such as pancreatitis, peritonitis, active or perfor-ated peptic ulcer, abdominal aortic aneurysm and gynaecological emergencies.

The severity of abdominal pain will govern the decision as to how soon a doctor should be seen.

Milder pain that occurs at some time during every day and persists for two weeks despite a course of antacids or analgesic requires referral if the symptoms are troublesome. Obviously, the presence of certain accompanying symptoms (see below) may shorten the period before a doc-tor should be seen.

Symptoms that do not occur on a daily basis may be left for a little longer, to assess the effect of symptomatic treatment, before referring to the doctor.

Type

Descriptions of the type of pain can be helpful to the diagnostician but they depend on the intelli-gence and articulacy of the patient.

Colic is a term used to describe waves of severe pain superimposed on a more constant duller pain and occurs when a hollow muscular organ is in spasm. Thus, a colicky or griping pain is most likely to indicate involvement of the stom-ach or bowel, the genito-urinary system (such as the ureter, bladder, uterus or fallopian tubes) or the bile duct system.

Abdominal pain will sometimes be described as a vague discomfort. This is typical of, but not exclusive to, the common indigestion seen with a non-specific gastritis. The condition is self-limiting, its cause usually being dietary overindulgence or poor eating habits.

A sharp burning sensation in the epigastric region or behind the sternum is typical of oesophagitis due to reflux, and is referred to as heartburn by the lay person. Such a sensation may also be caused by a peptic ulcer, although sometimes a patient with an ulcer will complain of a more specific gnawing pain that can be pointed to with a finger.

The pain of angina or a myocardial infarction can mimic oesophagitis and other causes of abdominal pain. Although these conditions will be seen relatively rarely in the pharmacy, they should always be borne in mind.

An inflammatory process in any organ in the abdomen may result in a sensation of tenderness over the affected area. It is therefore important to ask not only about pain but also about any tenderness, particularly when light pressure is applied with a finger or when the patient bends or stretches.

Onset

Factors surrounding the onset of abdominal pain can provide some useful clues about the diagnosis.

Pain related to meals generally indicates a lesion in the stomach or bowel and is a classic symptom of a peptic ulcer (as well as non-ulcerative inflammatory conditions of the gastric and bowel mucosa). Epigastric or central pain that occurs a few minutes after a meal is typical of gastric ulcer, while pain that occurs one to two hours after a meal is more typical of duodenal ulcer. The pain of a duodenal ulcer is usually worse during the night. Both of these types of pain may respond to antacids or H₂ antagonists, but pain that persists despite such treatment requires referral.

Pain or other abdominal symptoms following a single incident of overeating or excess alcohol may represent either a non-specific (or non-ulcer) gastritis or indigestion, which will resolve quickly without the need for referral. However, if symptoms become severe or persist, they could represent some underlying pathological cause, such as food poisoning.

Angina or myocardial infarction may be brought on by large meals. If this seems a possibility, it is important to establish whether the patient has a past history of ischaemic heart disease and also to bear in mind how ill the patient appears to be. Angina may also be brought on by the cold or exercise.

Any pain or discomfort that starts immediately on eating could represent oesophagitis or even a nervous dyspepsia. If simple OTC treatment is not successful, this condition requires attention and it is best to refer the patient for reassurance or investigation.

An acute hernia caused by lifting or straining may be felt as a severe pain in the groin or suprapubic region, while a muscle strain in the back may be referred to the lateral aspects of the loins, the hypochondria and the chest.

Severe pain or a throbbing or burning sensation on or after defaecation is typical of haemorrhoids but could also indicate anal fissure, fistula or rectal abscess. This type of pain requires referral.

Any abdominal injury or trauma with symptoms requires referral.

Abdominal symptoms such as pain, diarrhoea or constipation may be related to prescription drugs. Gastrointestinal symptoms can be caused by aspirin and other non-steroidal anti-inflammatory drugs (NSAIDs) and iron, while oesophageal symptoms may be caused by bulking agents, potassium salts, NSAIDs or tetracyclines, especially if the patient is lying in bed.

It is important to establish whether the onset of pain relates to the menstrual cycle. Mid-cycle pain may be caused by an ovulation syndrome while pain around the time of menstruation is likely to be due to some uterine spasm (such as dysmenorrhoea) or endometriosis.

Pain that occurs or is worse when the patient passes urine is likely to indicate cystitis or, less commonly, renal colic caused by a stone.

A sudden onset of abdominal pain, particularly in a previously fit individual, may well represent an acute abdomen, which has already been referred to.

Abdominal symptoms, especially indigestion or epigastric pain, that occur for the first time in a man of middle age or beyond and do not respond to simple antacids require referral, since gastric carcinoma is most common in males in this age group.

A sudden onset of chest symptoms, no matter how reminiscent they are of oesophagitis, should alert the pharmacist to consider the possibility of ischaemic heart disease and to question the patient further to exclude this possible diagnosis.

Accompanying symptoms

A large number of other symptoms may accompany abdominal pain or discomfort. They have been arranged here in approximate decreasing order of importance or severity.

Weight loss

Weight loss is a significant sign in anyone with abdominal symptoms and becomes more so with advancing years from middle age onwards. It may be caused by a peptic ulcer but it could signify a sinister pathology, such as a carcinoma, and should always be referred.

Blood in the stool

Melaena (blood in the stool) is a warning symptom that needs referral for either reassurance or investigation, particularly in the older population. If the patient gives a past history of haemorrhoids, it may be possible to differentiate spotting of blood on toilet tissue due to haemorrhoids from a black tarry stool containing blood from a lesion further up the bowel. However, if the symptoms have changed in a patient with previously diagnosed haemorrhoids or if there is any doubt whatsoever in the pharmacist's mind, then it is wise to refer the patient for a medical opinion.

Fresh (bright red) blood smearing the stool in a young person, associated with symptoms of haemorrhoids, is probably acceptable in the short term. However, above the age of 40 years old, any type of blood in the stool requires investigation.

Anaemia

The commonest cause of anaemia in patients admitted to hospital is a gastrointestinal bleed and it is therefore necessary to refer any patient with signs of anaemia, with or without abdominal symptoms, to the doctor.

Signs of anaemia are: tiredness, facial pallor, pale conjunctiva (seen by everting the lower eyelid and comparing with the red/pink conjunctiva lining the lower lid of a healthy person) and pale palms of the hands (again observed by comparing with the pink palms of a healthy individual). Severe anaemia may cause shortness of breath.

Menstrual disorders

Abdominal symptoms associated with specific times in the menstrual cycle, such as mid-cycle, premenstrual or perimenstrual pains, suggest that the problem relates to the genital tract. Where involvement of the genital tract is suspected or requires exclusion, any irregularity should be inquired for, such as a missed period, vaginal discharge, abnormal bleeding and particularly any symptoms associated with early pregnancy, such as nausea, breast changes and nocturia. Patients with pain associated with any of these features will generally require referral to exclude serious conditions such as a tubal pregnancy, salpingitis, or endometriosis.

Jaundice

Frank jaundice can be recognised by a yellow discoloration of the skin. More subtle signs can be detected by inspecting the sclera of the eye, which will have a yellow colour or tinge when compared with the white of a normal eye. Jaundice suggests liver or biliary involvement and requires referral.

Dysphagia

A genuine difficulty in swallowing food or drink requires prompt referral to exclude oesophageal obstruction. A feeling of a lump in the throat which does not affect swallowing should also be followed up, although perhaps not as urgently as genuine dysphagia.

Swelling

Localised swelling in the abdomen is associated with hernias. General abdominal distension may be real or imagined and can occur with relatively benign dyspepsia as well as with more serious diagnoses. However, referral is necessary if there is a real change in the abdominal girth measurement associated with abdominal symptoms.

More often, the patient will complain of feeling bloated, usually with flatulence. This is a common symptom of many abdominal disorders and is not really helpful in making a differential diagnosis.

Vomiting

Vomiting that persists for more than one or two days requires a medical opinion. Usually the cause will be food or alcohol intolerance or gastrointestinal infection, but it can occur as a result of severe pain (as in renal or biliary colic and appendicitis), in reflux oesophagitis and in nervous dyspepsia. In the presence of severe abdominal pain, vomiting may be a sign of obstruction.

Vomiting can also arise from extra-abdominal causes, such as migraine or a raised intracranial pressure.

In children, vomiting may be caused by fever, unassociated with other abdominal symptoms. This is common in acute systemic viral infections in the young. It is usually of no consequence, unless frequent enough to raise the possibility of dehydration or an alternative cause.

Diarrhoea and constipation

These two symptoms are considered in Chapters 6 and 7. Diarrhoea is often associated with abdominal colic and is common in gastroenteritis, diverticulitis and colitis. It may also occur with pain in appendicitis. In older patients, the pharmacist should be alert to the possibility of sinister causes.

Abdominal pain with constipation may be caused by a temporary impaction of the stool; if simple laxatives are not effective, the patient should be referred for exclusion of other causes of obstruction.

Dysuria/frequency

Pain or a burning sensation on passing urine, frequency and urgency may suggest a urinary tract infection or a renal stone. Inflammation of other organs in the abdomen, such as the bowel or appendix, can also irritate the urinary tract, causing these symptoms.

Rash

Severe pain on one side of the trunk is characteristic of herpes zoster infection (shingles), and often precedes the appearance of a rash. The rash follows the course of sensory nerves and may be seen across the front of the upper abdomen or chest, around the side of the trunk and on the back. The rash looks like that of chickenpox (flat at first, then forming pustules and vesicles). Immediate referral is necessary for the doctor to consider treatment with antiviral drugs, which should be started as early as possible after the diagnosis has been made.

Waterbrash

Waterbrash, the regurgitation of bitter gastric contents, is a common and not very specific symptom, which may occur in almost any kind of dyspepsia.

Aggravating and relieving factors

Pain from a peptic ulcer is not always aggravated by food; sometimes food acts as a buffer to the acid attacking the damaged mucosa and hence provides some relief. Classically, a gastric ulcer is said to be aggravated by food and a duodenal ulcer relieved by it.

Antacids and H_2 antagonists usually provide some relief in peptic ulceration and oesophagitis, whereas they do not help in nervous dyspepsia or in biliary colic due to gallstones. Pain in a patient with biliary colic due to gallstones will be exacerbated by fatty foods, and a reduction in the amount of fat eaten will relieve or prevent the pain to some degree. This is not always diagnostic in itself since the pain of peptic ulcer may be affected in the same way.

The pain of oesophagitis or acid reflux may be aggravated by lying down or bending over; sometimes smoking, alcohol, chocolate or coffee can lower the pressure in the oesophageal sphincter and allow reflux to take place.

The colicky pain of colitis or gastroenteritis will often be relieved temporarily by passing a stool, which differentiates these conditions from appendicitis in which no such relief will usually occur.

Pain caused by non-specific gastritis, peptic ulcer, oesophagitis or hiatus hernia can normally be relieved temporarily by antacids or H_2 antagonists. This may be helpful in distinguishing these conditions from angina. The pain of angina usually responds to sublingual glyceryl trinitrate, which may have been prescribed for the patient. Chest pain not responding to either type of drug should be evaluated in terms of the possibility of a myocardial infarction.

Special considerations in children

Abdominal pain in babies from the age of two weeks to four months may indicate colic. This usually occurs in the evenings. The baby will draw up its knees and will cry, despite being picked up. The condition resolves spontaneously by the age of four months.

One serious cause of abdominal pain in babies aged between four months and two years is intussusception. In this condition, two adjacent sections of bowel telescope together, causing obstruction and an acute abdomen. The condition is a medical emergency.

Projectile vomiting in babies at about six to eight weeks of age is a possible indicator of obstruction, such as pyloric stenosis. Referral is necessary.

Viral conditions can cause enlargement of the mesenteric lymph glands (in the abdomen) in children. This may produce a non-specific abdominal pain, usually associated with fever, which may be confused with other potentially more serious conditions. It usually resolves spontaneously.

Management

There are various lifestyle measures which patients with dyspepsia or reflux can take to give some symptomatic relief. Small, regular and frequent meals are better than hurried greasy food binges. Fat in food lowers the tone of the lower oesophageal sphincter, which is undesirable in acid reflux. Sphincter pressure may also be lowered by smoking, alcohol, chocolate, coffee, or even peppermint, which is present in some antacid preparations. Heartburn can often be relieved by raising the head of the bed and by avoiding bending and stooping.

Antacids

Antacid preparations are effective in providing symptomatic relief in dyspepsia and may be recommended as a first-line treatment. They should be taken one hour after meals for maximum efficacy. Earlier administration will result in the antacid being ejected from the stomach into the duodenum by gastric emptying, which normally occurs within an hour of eating. Also, food acts as a good buffer against acid attack on the gastric mucosa.

Although individual patients will state particular preferences for specific products, and *in vitro* tests have shown that some antacids are better than others in neutralising acid under laboratory conditions, it is probably true to say that OTC antacids are of similar clinical efficacy, provided that a large enough dose is taken. It is well established in the medical literature that reducing the acidity of the gastric contents gives symptomatic relief from dyspepsia, and at high doses traditional antacids are as effective as H_2 antagonists in relieving symptoms.

Table 8.2 Major drug interactions with antacids

Drug	Effect
Chlorpromazine	Reduced absorption
Ciprofloxacin, norfloxacin	Reduced absorption
Digoxin	Reduced absorption
Enteric-coated tablets	Coating disrupted in stomach
Iron	Reduced absorption
Lithium	Serum levels reduced by sodium (bicarbonate)
Penicillamine	Reduced absorption
Rifampicin	Reduced absorption
Sucralfate	Efficacy reduced as pH increases
Tetracyclines	Reduced absorption
Warfarin and phenindione	Reduced absorption

The most significant drug interactions with antacids are shown in Table 8.2.

If antacids do not give relief of symptoms or if the dosage is inconvenient to the patient, it will be appropriate, in the majority of cases, to consider the use of an H_2 antagonist. The H_2 antagonists cimetidine, famotidine and ranitidine are available OTC for the short-term relief of heartburn, dyspepsia and hyperacidity. They are very effective and should not be taken continuously for longer than two weeks without consulting a doctor, to avoid masking symptoms of serious disease. H_2 antagonists have a longer duration of action than antacids, have a convenient once-daily dosage, and are remarkably free of adverse effects. Because of its potential for drug interactions cimetidine should be avoided in patients taking phenytoin, theophylline and oral anticoagulants.

Magnesium salts

Magnesium salts are effective antacids but in doses required to give symptomatic relief they can cause diarrhoea.

Many products, for example magnesium carbonate mixture and magnesium trisilicate mixture, contain a relatively high sodium content, which may be unsuitable for patients with heart failure or hypertension.

Aluminium salts

Antacids containing aluminium are also effective. They are considered by some to be longer acting than magnesium salts because of a slowing effect on gut transit time. This, in turn, can lead to constipation in some patients. For this reason, they may be considered less suitable than magnesium salts for elderly patients.

Many proprietary antacids contain a mixture of aluminium and magnesium.

Calcium salts

Calcium salts have the reputation of being quick acting. They can lead to constipation and, theoretically at least, may cause acid rebound by stimulating secretion of gastrin, which in turn causes more acid to be secreted by the stomach. The clinical significance of this is unclear.

Bismuth salts

Bismuth is an old established antacid that is effective, but can cause constipation.

Sodium bicarbonate

Sodium bicarbonate is a fast-acting antacid but it should be avoided in patients whose sodium intake needs to be limited. It should not be used on a long-term basis since it is absorbed and may cause metabolic alkalosis.

Dimeticone

Dimeticone reduces the surface tension of the mucus-coated gas bubbles in the intestine so that small bubbles coalesce. It is claimed to act as a defoaming agent, allowing gas to be eliminated. It is included in many proprietary antacid mixtures.

Alginates

Alginates are present in some proprietary medicines and are useful for relieving symptoms of acid reflux into the oesophagus. They are said to form a floating viscous gel on top of the stomach contents. This protects the vulnerable mucous membrane of the oesophagus when the gastric contents are forced up into it. Such medicines are suitable for hiatus hernia and other causes of reflux.

It should be remembered that some mixtures containing alginates have relatively little acid-neutralising activity, as judged by the amount of antacid present, and are therefore inferior to other mixtures in this respect.

A combination of cimetidine and alginate is available for the treatment of heartburn.

Treatment strategy by the doctor

Various consensus guidelines exist for the management of ulcer-like dyspepsia and reflux in primary care and pharmacists should be aware of the strategies of local general practitioners so as to be able to educate and reassure their patients.

Generally, in patients under 45 years old with significant dyspepsia, the possibility of a peptic ulcer, whose symptoms persist after treatment with antacids or H_2 antagonists, should be suggested and a test for *Helicobacter pylori* may be performed. Those with a positive test result will usually be prescribed *H. pylori* eradication treatment and those with a negative result will usually be prescribed an ulcer healing drug. Patients aged 45 years and over, as well as all patients with significant accompanying symptoms such as vomiting, weight loss, fullness, difficulty in swallowing, loss of appetite or taking NSAIDs may be considered for endoscopic investigation.

Similar guidelines exist for the treatment of patients with symptoms of gastro-oesophageal reflux disease. Patients over 45 years or with significant accompanying symptoms will be considered for endoscopy and those under 45 will usually be treated with either an H_2 antagonist or a proton pump inhibitor.

Spasmolytic drugs

Drugs that relax smooth muscle can relieve certain abdominal symptoms. Loperamide is a useful antidiarrhoeal agent and was mentioned in the earlier chapter on diarrhoea. It will give some relief of intestinal colic associated with diarrhoea.

Dicyclomine (dicycloverine), alverine and hyoscine are antispasmodic drugs and are suitable for the treatment of gastrointestinal colic (the products differ in their recommendations for minimum age of use). Hyoscine is also licensed for use in primary dysmenorrhoea (i.e. dysmenorrhoea that is not secondary to another condition).

Anticholinergics, such as hyoscine and dicyclomine (dicycloverine), may cause dryness of the mouth, some blurring of vision and palpitations. They are contraindicated in patients with glaucoma or prostatitis.

Analgesics and NSAIDs

Analgesics can be used for relief of abdominal pain. Aspirin is best avoided because of its irritant effect on the gastrointestinal tract.

Ibuprofen can be useful for the relief of dysmenorrhoea and other pain associated with the genital tract in women.

 SUMMARY OF CONDITIONS PRODUCING ABDOMINAL PAIN

Acute abdomen

Acute abdomen is the term used to describe a potentially life-threatening situation. Because of the severity of the illness, the patient will not present to the pharmacy but a relative may describe the symptoms. The patient will have severe pain of sudden recent onset, be obviously ill, have abdominal tenderness and will lie still because movement will cause more pain. There may be fever, vomiting and abdominal distension. Causes include peritonitis, bowel infarction, bowel obstruction, pancreatitis, abdominal aortic aneurysm and gynaecological emergencies – **refer** urgently.

Abdominal aortic aneurysm

An aneurysm is a localised, abnormal dilatation of a blood vessel. In the abdominal aorta this is often due to an atheroslerotic/ageing process. The aneurysm weakens the wall of the aorta, which may rupture. Symptoms are abdominal pain, usually epigastric, radiating to the back, and a pulsating mass may be felt in the abdomen. It is a medical emergency – **refer.**

Appendicitis

An inflamed appendix may occur at any age but is relatively rare in babies. It presents as pain that is central or in the right iliac fossa, often moving from the former to the latter region within a few hours of onset. The pain is continuous and there is right-sided tenderness. The pain may be accompanied by vomiting and either diarrhoea or constipation related to inflammation of the surrounding bowel – **refer.**

Biliary colic

Spasm of the common bile duct may be caused by obstruction of the duct by gallstones or by infection of the biliary network. It presents as abdominal pain, epigastric, central but often high in the right hypochondrium and is also felt in the back and in the tips of the shoulders. There is often nausea and vomiting – **refer.**

Carcinoma

Carcinoma of the oesophagus occurs mostly in adults over 50 years old. There is a period of silent growth before the appearance of symptoms (food lodging in the oesophagus, loss of weight and sometimes pain on swallowing).

→

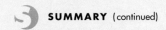 **SUMMARY** (continued)

Carcinoma of the stomach causes few symptoms until the growth of the tumour is advanced and the prognosis is usually poor at the time of diagnosis. Although it sometimes occurs in patients with a long history of indigestion, it often arises in patients without previous symptoms. The peak incidence is between 40 and 60 years of age and it is more common in men than women. The patient will complain of indigestion at first and later pain on a daily basis with loss of weight and vomiting. Although anti-ulcer therapy may give some relief for a few weeks, the patient eventually deteriorates.

Cancer of the large bowel or colon is slow growing and is potentially curable if diagnosed early. It presents as a change in bowel habit in patients beyond middle age, with abdominal pain, distension and blood or mucus in the stool.

Cancer of the rectum usually presents as diarrhoea, with blood present, but occasionally it may present as constipation. There is abdominal discomfort and pain in the rectum with loss of weight. Rectal tumours vary considerably in their rate of growth – **refer**.

Diverticular disease
Diverticulitis produces a colicky pain. The pain may last from one to three days and then settles and is followed by a symptom-free period before recurring. It may be accompanied by diarrhoea and blood in the stool, or by constipation – **refer**. See also Chapter 6.

Dysmenorrhoea
Dysmenorrhoea presents as severe pain around the time of menstruation and is caused by uterine spasm. Primary dysmenorrhoea usually occurs in younger women whereas secondary dysmenorrhoea, which is associated with an underlying condition, such as fibroids or endometriosis, can occur in older women too. The pain is either colicky or dull, usually in the lower abdomen, and often radiating to the back. It starts either a few days or hours before menstruation and ceases one or two days after menstruation begins. Mild cases may respond to NSAIDs such as ibuprofen, but if persistent or severe – **refer**.

Endometriosis
Endometriosis is the abnormal presence of endometrial tissue at sites outside the uterus. The abnormal sites are usually located in the abdomen, and include the peritoneum, ovary, bladder and intestines. It is a cause of dysmenorrhoea (see above) and can also cause pelvic inflammation and infertility – **refer**.

Gastritis and gastroenteritis
Irritation leading to inflammation of the mucosa of the stomach or small bowel, giving variable and often diffuse abdominal pain or indigestion, is often caused by overindulgence in either food or alcohol. Vomiting may also be present. It is often referred to as non-specific gastritis or non-ulcer dyspepsia (in which the cause is undiagnosed) and resolves spontaneously within one or two days. In children, non-specific gastritis is associated with fever. Other causes of gastritis or gastroenteritis include bacterial contaminants in food (food poisoning), viruses (gastric flu) and protozoal infections in travellers from abroad. If the condition does not respond to rest, fluids and simple OTC measures within a few days – **refer**.

Hernias
Abdominal hernias are caused by a weakening of the muscles and supporting tissue in the abdomen, which allows protrusion (herniation) of the contents. They are common in the lower parts of the abdomen, where structures leave the abdominal cavity. They are often brought on by lifting or straining. The

(continued overleaf)

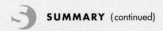 **SUMMARY** (continued)

commonest types are inguinal hernias (where the spermatic cord leaves the abdomen) and femoral hernias (where femoral vessels leave the abdomen). The former, seen in males, presents as a swelling in the suprapubic area, which eventually pushes into the scrotum. It is felt as an ache in the groin. Femoral hernias occur in both sexes and may be felt as a colicky pain. The swelling is small. Umbilical hernias, with protrusion of the umbilicus, are common in babies. They are usually of no consequence and in most cases resolve as the baby grows – **refer**.

Hiatus hernia

Hiatus hernia is a weakness at the oesophageal hiatus (where the oesophagus penetrates the diaphragm) such that the lower oesophagus and/or part of the stomach is able to slide up through the diaphragm into the chest. The oblique entry of the oesophagus into the stomach disappears and reflux of gastric contents into the oesophagus readily occurs. Hiatus hernia may be congenital, but more usually develops in later life. It occurs also when there is an increase in intra-abdominal pressure, as in obesity or pregnancy. Hiatus hernia is sometimes asymptomatic but generally produces heartburn, which can be treated with antacids. Surgery is occasionally required to rectify the abnormality – **refer**.

Inflammatory bowel disease

See Chapter 7. Abdominal pain is usually mild, the main symptom being bloody diarrhoea. A colicky pain may precede a bowel motion – **refer**.

Irritable bowel syndrome

See Chapter 7.

Nervous dyspepsia

The main symptoms of nervous dyspepsia (functional gastritis) are pain and vomiting. Psychological causes, such as tension or anxiety, are usually easily found.

Non-ulcer (non-specific) gastritis/dyspepsia

In this condition there is inflammation of the gastric mucosa caused by smoking, NSAIDs, alcohol or of no known cause, whereas in gastric ulcer, gastritis may follow or precede the development of a crater or ulcer in the gastric wall.

Oesophagitis

Oesophagitis commonly occurs either as a result of a primary inflammatory lesion in the oesophagus or as a result of reflux, when the lower oesophageal sphincter fails to prevent the gastric contents entering the oesophagus when the patient lies flat. Oesophagitis is a common symptom in peptic and oesophageal ulceration and hiatus hernia.

→

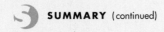

Pancreatitis

See also biliary colic. Pancreatitis is an inflammatory condition of the pancreas, commonly caused by gallstones, alcohol, infection or tumours. It causes sudden acute abominal pain, as described under biliary colic and acute abdomen – **refer**.

Peptic ulcer

Peptic ulcers destroy the mucosa and submucosal tissues of the stomach and duodenum. Their first occurrence is most common in males under 35 years of age. The chief symptom is abdominal pain, usually epigastric, but sometimes in the right hypochondrium in duodenal ulcer. Pain is relieved by simple antacids as well as H_2 antagonists and prescribed proton pump inhibitors. The onset of pain is related to food. It may occur either soon after a meal (gastric ulcer) or one to two hours after a meal (duodenal ulcer). Alternatively, food may relieve the pain. The pain of duodenal ulcer is often worse at night and when a meal is delayed or missed. Other symptoms include heartburn, waterbrash, belching and abdominal distension. If untreated, there may be perforation of the ulcer, bleeding and anaemia – **refer**.

Reflux oesophagitis (gastro-oesophageal reflux disease)

In this condition there is inflammation of the oesophagus caused by regurgitation of food, acid and bile into the lower oesophagus from the stomach. It is usually caused by a reduction in tone of the lower oesophageal sphincter in predisposed individuals.

Renal colic

Renal colic is usually caused by a renal stone blocking a ureter. There is severe pain in one loin, which may initially start as an ache. The pain then spreads down the flank and into the suprapubic region or, in males, the scrotum. The episode of pain may last several hours and will recur at intervals of days or weeks as the stone passes down the urinary tract. There will often be blood in the urine. Vomiting may occur because of the intense pain – **refer**.

Salpingitis

Salpingitis, an acute form of pelvic inflammatory disease, is a relatively rare condition in which there is inflammation of the fallopian tubes caused by infection. The condition produces lower abdominal pain, tenderness in the iliac fossa and usually a fever. A pregnancy in the fallopian tube (ectopic pregnancy) may be suspected if there is pain, often with bleeding, following eight to 10 weeks of amenorrhoea – **refer**.

Urinary tract infection

Pain (usually a burning pain on passing urine), frequency and urgency are symptoms of a urinary tract infection. Infection is most common in the bladder (cystitis). There may be fever and suprapubic pain and tenderness. Recurrences are common, particularly in women. The condition is less common in men and unusual in children, and should be referred. In women, individual mild cases will resolve spontaneously but if the patient has frequent recurrences – **refer**.

WHEN TO REFER
Abdominal disorders

• Sudden onset of intense pain that does not abate	Immediate referral
• Symptoms related to medication	
• Pain unrelated to meals	
• Persistent pain, not responding to OTC medication	
• Age over 45	
• Blood in stool	
• Weight loss	
• Dysphagia	
• Swelling (not bloating)	
• Vomiting for more than one to two days	
• Diarrhoea or constipation for more than one week	
• Anaemia	
• Jaundice	Immediate referral
• Dysuria	
• Aggravated by exercise or effort	Immediate referral
• Pain radiates to arm, neck or jaw	Immediate referral
• Pain radiates to back	
• Pain radiates to testis or suprapubic region	Immediate referral
• Pain radiates from central region to right iliac fossa	Immediate referral

CASE STUDIES

Case 1

A fit-looking couple in their 60s, not regular visitors to the pharmacy, ask to speak to 'the senior pharmacist'. The man wishes to purchase an antacid or one of the stronger medicines he has seen advertised on the television. His wife stands behind him saying nothing.

The request arises from infrequent indigestion, nothing serious, but annoying. On questioning, the man's answers become vague and his wife becomes agitated. Finally, the pharmacist asks directly whom the medicine is for, and the wife steps forward. She has suffered from dyspeptic symptoms for over two months, often after food and often at night. Her diet is good, she has never smoked and only drinks alcohol occasionally, but she looks unwell and rather pale. She has lost weight recently.

When the pharmacist suggests that no recommendation should be made but that the woman should see her doctor she becomes more agitated and her husband somewhat angry. To calm the situation they all agree reluctantly on a short-term H_2 antagonist and an early doctor's appointment.

The pharmacist remains worried, and is relieved to see the husband again about a week later, although he is still tense. He produces a prescription for the same medication, although this time for a

→

month, as a triumph. The doctor clearly knows best, he says, and has suggested there may even be a better medication that can be prescribed when a few investigations have been done. The pharmacist enquires further about the wife's health and progress, but the answers are evasive. The prescription is filled, the conversation ended.

A month passes before the woman herself appears. She still looks underweight, but vastly more cheerful, and has a prescription, this time for *Helicobacter* eradication therapy. She is more than happy to explain. So worried were they that an urgent private appointment was made with a gastroenterologist, who promptly performed endoscopy and biopsy. The findings were of non-ulcer dyspepsia, moderate reflux, and of course the infection. Both she and her husband were terrified of cancer, and cannot apologise enough for their behaviour. However, all is well, and the pharmacist discusses with her the immediate therapy, a subsequent acid suppressant regime and the probable need for intermittent treatment thereafter.

Case 2

On this occasion the pharmacist is at home in the evening, when friends telephone. They have just returned from holiday in the Mediterranean and had arranged dinner for the following evening. The trip was excellent, although on one occasion the man had got up at night to go to the toilet and found his urine bright pink. However, there had been no pain, and as they had enjoyed a large restaurant meal that evening they dismissed the incident as due to exotic ingredients in the food. With time it was even possible to wonder if it were all imagined.

The dinner the next evening passes pleasantly, although it is marred in part when the friend declines to eat, again blaming the holiday diet and asking the pharmacist for advice. It is agreed he should rest his stomach, with just water overnight at least. With this he retires to bed early.

The next afternoon his wife calls in at the pharmacy. Her husband is now in hospital. He suffered increasing and eventually severe abdominal pain during the night, the worst he has ever known. The doctor came in the early hours, and gave a pethidine injection. He settled for a while, but the pain returned in the early morning and he was admitted.

After closing the pharmacy that evening the pharmacist visits the hospital and is relieved to find his friend more comfortable. X-rays and scans have revealed a renal stone low down in the ureter, for which he is receiving adequate pain relief. The original discoloured urine was probably the start of it. The calculus must have been there for some time, but the Mediterranean heat and abundant alcohol used to counter it may have provoked a degree of dehydration, and in turn renal colic. He is grateful to have arrived home first. The next day the offending item was removed via a cystoscope, and a short while afterwards he was restored to normal activity, with the possible exception of his intake of wine.

Case 3

It is satisfying to make, or suspect, a diagnosis, but sometimes it is much more important just to respond to the almost subconscious feeling that something is wrong.

A pleasant man in his late 60s, well known to his pharmacist, visits fairly regularly for his repeat prescription for mild and well-controlled hypertension, and the occasional self-medication. On one occasion it is an antacid, the next time paracetamol for a headache. After that he seeks advice for diarrhoea, and remembering the previous history he is advised to seek medical advice. He does so willingly, although by the time of the appointment the diarrhoea has stopped and a clinical examination is normal.

The man has a further small quantity of paracetamol, and returns later to buy a stronger analgesic, a

(continued overleaf)

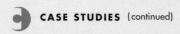

codeine combination. The pharmacist enquires. This is for recurrent, although not severe, abdominal pain, and when at the surgery for a blood pressure check he was advised this might help his pain and the occasional looseness in the bowel more effectively.

Two months later his wife calls for a further supply. The most recent episode has left him in bed, getting better now, but without medication. The pharmacist is unhappy as there has now been a long history of vague central abdominal pain, in episodes, feeling well in between. The man's hypertension remains reasonably controlled, and he usually sees the practice nurse. He does have occasional bowel upsets, but likes a can or more of beer in the evenings, which perhaps explains not only that but his moderate obesity as well. Although it is difficult to be specific, the pharmacist feels uneasy, and knowing him to be compliant, suggests a doctor's appointment next time specifically to look at these problems.

Often such suspicions come to nothing. With this man, a series of blood and urine tests, as well as an X-ray, were reported normal and he was extremely fortunate to have an ultrasound scan. The aneurysm thus discovered was resected and grafted urgently, and it was noted at the time of the operation that a number of minor leaks into and through its wall had already occurred.

9

Perianal and perivulval pruritus

Pruritus in the genitalia and in the perianal region is a minor symptom that can be treated with OTC medicines, provided that certain criteria are met. The symptom is relatively common but because patients may be embarrassed to discuss it, some will self-diagnose and medicate without consulting a pharmacist. Many of the common conditions that give rise to pruritus are recurrent and it is important that patients are educated and advised appropriately. Inappropriate or prolonged medication might exacerbate the condition or mask some underlying pathology.

Common conditions

The most common conditions that cause perianal and perivulval itch are cystitis or urethritis, vulvovaginitis (from infection of the vagina, most commonly with yeasts or bacteria, haemorrhoids (piles) and threadworm (pinworm) infestation.

Assessing symptoms

Site or location

Although the symptoms of haemorrhoids and threadworm are easily located to the perianal region, there may be some overlap in the symptoms of vulvovaginal infection and cystitis in women. This is in part because of the close proximity of the vulva and the urethral opening, but also because of irritation of the vulva in cystitis caused by urine dripping from the urethra. It is

of course important to locate the site of pruritus to differentiate cystitis from vaginitis. This is sometimes difficult to do.

Presence of a rash on the perivulval skin may be caused by sensitisation to toiletries, synthetic underwear or the use of products containing local anaesthetics.

Type and severity of symptoms

Vaginal candidiasis (thrush) usually presents as vulval soreness, itching and a burning sensation in the vulval area. There is often redness or swelling of the vulva and a thick, white, odourless discharge. By contrast the discharge of bacterial vaginitis is smelly and offensive.

Although less common in men, thrush can cause itching, burning and/or redness at the tip of the penis or under the foreskin. A burning sensation is felt on urinating. A penile discharge is best referred to exclude a sexually transmitted disease (STD).

Patients with cystitis (usually women) will complain of itching at the exit of the urethra. Cystitis in men is much rarer, and should be referred for investigation. A burning sensation will be described when passing urine (dysuria). Patients may also complain of urinary frequency and urgency. Rarely, loin pain will be felt. In such cases, the infection may have ascended into the kidney and the patient should be referred.

Patients with mild cases of haemorrhoids, or in the early stages of the condition, will complain of itching in the perianal region. More severely affected patients, especially those with external haemorrhoids, may suffer intense pain. Anal fistulae or fissures in the anal canal are also painful. Any patient complaining of pain should be referred for examination and an accurate diagnosis.

Threadworm causes itching around the anus, particularly at night. This may produce acute pain in some children, particularly when scratching has caused excoriation of the skin in the perianal area.

Onset

Infections of the vagina can be a complication or accompany a course of antibiotics or steroids. Pregnancy predisposes to an overgrowth of *Candida* and some experts believe that the use of oral contraceptives may alter the vaginal environment and cause candidiasis. Pregnancy or suspected pregnancy requires referral. Diabetes is another predisposing factor for candidiasis.

In cases of vaginal candidiasis, patients should be asked about use of local topical applications, such as vaginal deodorants or bath additives, as these can predispose or exacerbate the condition.

Sexual intercourse can cause trauma, with a resulting urethritis. This gives rise to the well-known condition of honeymoon cystitis.

A patient may relate the onset of haemorrhoids to a cough, sneeze or episode of physical exertion. They may first appear when straining at stool, or during episodes of constipation.

Symptoms of threadworm infestation have a sudden onset, commonly at night-time. This is because the eggs are laid by the female worms at night when the environment is warm. Scratching by the patient causes the female worms to rupture, liberating more eggs. The pruritus is associated with some factor or chemical in the eggs.

Dysuria, frequency, vaginitis, discharge, urethritis and rashes in the genital region are all possible symptoms of STD and may occur within a few days of sexual intercourse with an infected partner. STDs will not present frequently to pharmacists but it is important to regard symptoms associated with such a time-scale with a high index of suspicion, especially in young adults, the single, those returning from holiday or whose job involves a lot of travel, and indi-

viduals (or their partners) who have been treated previously for STD. There are frequently concerns about the possibility of HIV infection, when no symptoms will be evident. These should be handled sensitively, explaining the low probability amongst heterosexuals, the need for safe sex and that the antibody blood test will not be accurate until three months from exposure. Referral for counselling is recommended.

Duration and frequency

Most patients will seek relief of symptoms promptly. Vaginal candidiasis may be treated with topical OTC imidazoles for one week or with an oral imidazole as a single dose. If there is no obvious improvement after one week, the patient should be referred to exclude other conditions. Referral should also be made if the patient has suffered from similar symptoms on more than two previous occasions in the past six months, so that any underlying predisposing condition, such as diabetes, can be identified and a differential diagnosis made to exclude other diseases.

If the patient is known to have diabetes and has recurrent episodes of candidiasis she should be questioned about the control of her diabetes and referred if appropriate.

Mild cases of cystitis usually resolve spontaneously within a few days. Symptoms that persist beyond three days require referral so that antibiotic treatment can be considered. As with candidiasis, frequent recurrence may suggest that the patient has some predisposing condition, such as diabetes, or an anatomical or physiological abnormality in the urinary tract. Changes in the urethral and vaginal epithelium at the menopause may increase the likelihood of infection in some women; in such cases, local application of oestrogen may be helpful. If symptoms are recurrent around the time of menstruation in younger women and do not respond to OTC medicines, the patient should be assessed by a doctor.

Thrush can be a chronic complaint and patients may complain of a discharge for several weeks. A long-standing discharge, however, is unlikely to be vaginitis, and is more often associated with pelvic inflammatory disease, hormonal disturbance or other systemic illness.

Patients with threadworm will usually seek help within a few days of symptoms occurring. They can be treated at any stage of the disease with OTC anthelmintics, provided that there is no reason for referral. Initial treatment may be followed with a repeat dose 14 days later (see Management). Any cases that have not resolved within a few days or which recur after two weeks require special consideration for referral or counselling on prophylactic measures.

Mild cases of haemorrhoids may not present to pharmacists or doctors for a long time after the condition first becomes symptomatic. Ideally, any rectal bleeding requires a diagnosis by a doctor, especially in middle aged and elderly patients, to exclude any serious cause. However, if bleeding is noted just as spotting or streaks on the toilet paper after defaecation, and there is only a mild pruritus, OTC medication and advice will usually be appropriate, at least for a short time, if the patient is reticent about seeing a doctor.

Haemorrhoids can often recur. Aggravating factors, such as constipation, can sometimes be identified and it is important that these are dealt with as well as the haemorrhoids themselves.

Accompanying symptoms

Vaginal candidiasis

In this condition there is often (but not always) a characteristic vaginal discharge, which is usually described as thick and white or creamy (resembling cottage cheese) but odourless. However, the discharge can sometimes be thin and watery or yellow in colour; this type of discharge is also typical of some other vaginal infections, which may not respond to topical imidazoles and require referral for investigation.

A thin, watery discharge in a postmenopausal woman may be due to candidal infection. However, referral is necessary if the condition does not respond to OTC imidazoles so that atrophic vaginitis and carcinoma can be excluded.

The discharge associated with candidiasis is odourless. Any offensive smelly discharge requires referral since it may represent a trichomonal or bacterial infection. Similarly, blood-stains in the discharge or any bleeding not associated with menstruation should be referred to exclude a sinister cause. A slight discharge is normal in some women and reassurance is all that is needed, provided that the discharge has not changed in any way, such as amount, smell or texture, and is not irritant or bloodstained.

Other symptoms in a patient with vulvovaginitis that should be regarded as unusual and require referral include vaginal blisters, abdominal pain, fever, vomiting and diarrhoea. These may indicate other local pathology or pelvic inflammation. Dyspareunia (painful intercourse) may be caused by candidiasis but could indicate other pathology. The patient should be referred for a full examination and assessment. If the patient is pregnant, receiving immunosuppressive drugs or is known to have HIV infection, referral is necessary. The popular belief that oral contraceptives may predispose to vaginal candidiasis remains controversial. However, if candidiasis is recurrent, patients taking oral contraceptives may be referred so that the doctor can assess the value of trying a different pill. Referral should also be made if the patient, or their partner, has a known history of STD so that both partners can be treated and relapses prevented.

Any patient with symptoms lasting more than seven days despite treatment should be referred. This is because the differential diagnosis can be difficult and conditions such as STD, bacterial infection, trichomoniasis, genital herpes and warts may present with similar (although often more severe) soreness, inflammation and oedema.

Cystitis

If the symptoms of dysuria and frequency are accompanied by pain in the loins, with or without vomiting (suggesting infection or other conditions high in the urinary tract), fever or blood in the urine (indicating more severe infection or inflammation), the patient should be referred.

The urine may be turbid or smell 'fishy' and

this may cause no concern on its own, unless persistent. However, if the symptoms of cystitis or urethritis are accompanied by a vaginal discharge, then it is wise to refer the patient.

Pregnant women often present with the symptoms of cystitis. These may represent nothing more than the mechanical effects of pressure from an enlarging uterus and will often resolve spontaneously in a few days. However, if symptoms are either persistent or recurrent, the patient should be referred.

Urinary frequency is a presenting feature of diabetes. If this symptom has lasted for more than a few days, is marked at night and is accompanied by thirst and weight loss, the patient should be referred.

Patients who are known diabetics should present no special problems unless any of the referrable symptoms above are described. However, the patient should be advised to keep a close watch on blood glucose concentrations since a return of symptoms may indicate hyperglycaemia.

Cystitis is rare in young men. It may be a manifestation of a renal stone, causing damage and infection in the renal tract. In such cases, the patient will complain of episodes of severe colicky loin pain spreading downwards, over days or longer, to the groin and the testicles. It requires a medical appraisal. Referral is also necessary if there is a penile discharge or a known history of STD.

In older men, cystitis is more common but referral is needed for exclusion of prostatic disease and bladder neoplasms. Blood in the urine, hesitancy on starting urination, a weak flow or dribbling of urine are all signs for referral.

Threadworm

In a child, perianal itching that is worse at night will almost certainly be caused by threadworm. The diagnosis is clinched by finding the small white worms, which measure 5 to 10 mm in length, either in the stool or, very occasionally, on the skin between the buttocks.

Perianal itching in adults, in the absence of a family history of threadworm or visual confirmation of worm infestation, may be due to irritation by deodorants, tight nylon underclothes or

to the other causes of perianal and perivulval itch considered in this chapter.

Scratching of the perianal area can cause the skin to become inflamed and sometimes broken. If this is troublesome, the patient should be referred to exclude infection or dermatitis, both of which will be resistant to treatment.

Persistent or particularly heavy cases of threadworm in children can cause loss of appetite, weight loss, insomnia and irritability. Such cases should be referred. Migrating worms have been said to cause inflammation of the vulva and vagina, causing itching and discharge.

Haemorrhoids

Constipation can cause or aggravate haemorrhoids.

Blood in the stool is common in patients with haemorrhoids and this is well known by most lay people. Since the vast majority of patients will not consult their doctor about mild cases of haemorrhoids, it is easy for them to become blasé about this symptom. Although the correct advice is to refer all patients with rectal bleeding who have not received a diagnosis from a doctor, some patients with mild haemorrhoids are likely to prefer to self-diagnose. Since blood in the stool can signify serious disease, some working guidelines are appropriate. These, of course, depend on the patient being able to give a clear description of their symptoms.

Fresh blood coating the stool is typical of lesions in the descending colon and rectum, and patients with this symptom should be referred to exclude serious pathology. Similarly, any blood that is evident in the flush water in the toilet requires referral. Blood mixed in the stool, giving a dark red or black tarry appearance, suggests that the source is higher in the gastrointestinal tract. This is typical of bleeding gastric or duodenal ulcers or lesions such as polyps or cancers in the colon. Such cases should be referred.

If blood is present as spots or streaks on the toilet paper, accompanying other symptoms of haemorrhoids, referral for a medical opinion may not be necessary, provided that no severe pain, diarrhoea, loss of appetite, nausea or vomiting have occurred and the pruritus is mild. However, if there is any doubt, referral should be made, especially in middle-aged and elderly patients in whom colorectal cancer is relatively more common.

Conditions that require referral, and may be suspected if there is severe pain, include a thrombosed haemorrhoid (when a prolapsing varicoele strangulates and clots) and various infections such as a perianal abscess or Bartholin's abscess (an infection of a fluid-secreting gland opening into the vagina), or an anal fissure or fistula.

Aggravating factors

Various factors that can initiate or predispose to perivulval and perianal pruritus have been referred to already. Symptoms can be aggravated by the following factors.

Passing urine will cause a burning sensation or other discomfort in cystitis and also in some cases of vulvovaginitis, such as candidiasis, when urine dribbles onto the sensitive area.

Constipation will aggravate haemorrhoids, and the symptoms of haemorrhoids are usually worse after a bowel motion.

Perfumed soaps, bubble bath, locally applied deodorants, and disinfectants may aggravate an already sensitive skin or mucosa caused by any of the conditions described above, producing pruritus and vaginitis.

Tampons and intrauterine contraceptive devices may aggravate vaginal candidiasis as may menstruation and sexual intercourse.

Tight underclothing made from synthetic material, such as nylon tights, will increase the temperature and humidity of the perianal and perivulval region, thus fostering ideal conditions for growth of bacteria and candida, as well as encouraging the female threadworm to lay eggs. Nightclothes and bedding will create a similar warm environment.

Hot baths also aggravate symptoms of pruritus.

OTC products advertised for the treatment of 'embarrassing itching', and which contain local anaesthetic agents, such as benzocaine, can sensitise perianal and perivulval skin, thus aggravating rather than relieving the condition.

Special considerations

Age

Children under 16 years of age should be referred if they have any of the symptoms described in this chapter, except for threadworm, since such symptoms are rare in this age group. Any suspicion of child abuse or of sexual intercourse under the age of 16 years should be handled delicately and diplomatically; but in every case the doctor, health visitor or social worker should be informed. Confidentiality should be respected whenever possible, although the interests of the child at risk are paramount.

Since the incidence of cancer increases with age, OTC treatment should not be recommended in the elderly if there is any doubt about the diagnosis. For instance, vaginal candidiasis is rare in women over 60 years of age and symptoms suggesting such a diagnosis should therefore be referred for confirmation.

Males

In older patients (from middle age onwards) the possibility of prostatitis should be considered if perineal pain with hesitancy and dysuria is present.

In younger men, cystitis is relatively uncommon compared with women and any symptoms suggesting this condition should be referred either to the general practitioner or, in cases where an STD is suspected, to the local genito-urinary out-patient clinic.

Patients with suspected STD

Any patient with a history of STD or with a partner suspected of having an STD is best advised to consult the local genito-urinary out-patient clinic for rapid diagnosis and treatment. Pharmacists should reassure patients that they will be dealt with in a friendly, confidential, anonymous and professional manner.

Management

Threadworm

Treatment of threadworm itself is relatively simple but compliance with additional hygienic measures is necessary to prevent reinfestation.

Mebendazole and piperazine are both available as single-dose OTC treatments for threadworm. All family members should be treated to obtain the maximal effect, even if they are asymptomatic.

Piperazine is presented as a powder that should be dissolved in water or milk. The initial dose should be followed by a second dose 14 days later to kill the worms that hatched from eggs present at the time that the first dose was taken. Piperazine should not be recommended for patients with epilepsy or in pregnancy. The powder can be used in children over three months. Piperazine elixir is taken daily for seven days, repeated after one week if necessary. For children under two it should be used on medical advice only.

Mebendazole is suitable for children over two years old. It is contraindicated in pregnancy. It is available as a chewable tablet and is effective often without the need to repeat the dose after 14 days, although this is a sensible precaution, as with piperazine. Parents of children with threadworm should be reassured that it is a common condition, is harmless and, despite the stigma once attached to it, does not reflect poor hygiene or diet.

Various measures should be taken to break the cycle of re-infestation, otherwise any recommended medicine may fail to have a lasting effect. Bed linen and towels should be washed frequently and underwear and nightclothes changed daily. Hands should be washed and nails scrubbed before eating and after going to the toilet to reduce transmission of eggs from anus to mouth. Airborne transmission is also possible and since eggs will be found in dust on floors and furniture, thorough vacuuming may be helpful. A bath or shower taken early in the morning helps to remove eggs laid overnight. Some patients may not obtain instant relief of symptoms after use of an anthelmintic. In such cases, crotamiton cream has been suggested to be useful as an adjuvant to treatment.

Cystitis

Symptomatic relief from cystitis is commonly achieved by drinking plenty of fluids and taking sodium bicarbonate (5 g every three to four hours), sodium citrate or potassium citrate to alkalinise the urine.

Patient counselling can include advice to empty the bladder as completely as possible after urinating and to avoid delay in emptying the bladder. Perianal hygiene is important and patients should be encouraged to wash the area with water and unperfumed soap after a bowel movement and to wipe from front to back to prevent re-infection.

If symptoms are related to intercourse, the perianal skin should be washed beforehand and the bladder should be emptied before and after intercourse. A lubricant should be used to prevent trauma and soreness.

Care should be taken to avoid tight underclothes made of synthetic material. Detergents should be thoroughly rinsed out after washing underclothes.

Cautions regarding the use of OTC cystitis products are outlined in Table 9.1.

Haemorrhoids

OTC treatments for haemorrhoids are available as suppositories, creams and ointments. Most contain mixtures of astringents (bismuth salts), local anaesthetics, antiseptics, antipruritics, zinc and other miscellaneous substances. However, the most effective preparation is likely to be one that contains hydrocortisone, a proven anti-inflammatory agent. Local anaesthetics should only be used for short periods because of the risk of sensitisation of the skin.

Patients who are constipated should be advised that this will exacerbate the symptoms of haemorrhoids. They should be recommended a laxative for the short term and counselled about adding more roughage (or bran) to the diet and increasing liquid intake. Bulking agents,

Table 9.1 Contraindications and need for care in the use of potassium- and sodium-containing preparations

Contraindication	Need for care
Renal disease	Patients may have impaired ability to excrete potassium in potassium citrate
	Effervescent products can cause accumulation of aluminium in renal patients taking aluminium salts as a phosphate binder
Pregnancy, hypertensive patients	Caution with extra sodium intake with sodium bicarbonate and citrate
Patients taking ACE inhibitors or potassium-sparing diuretics	Potassium citrate may cause hyperkalaemia
Patients taking nitrofurantoin	Nitrofurantoin is inactivated in alkaline urine
Patients taking lithium	Sodium salts can reduce plasma lithium levels

such as ispaghula and sterculia, are suitable, but if constipation has been present for some time, or is particularly stubborn, a stimulant laxative such as senna may be appropriate to obtain the first motion.

Pregnant women who suffer from haemorrhoids should be advised to increase the fibre content of their diet, since the high progesterone levels in pregnancy have the effect of relaxing the smooth muscle of the bowel.

The cornerstone of relieving the symptoms of haemorrhoids is perianal hygiene. The perianal skin should be washed at least once daily, and then patted dry, to prevent irritation by faecal matter in the perianal folds.

Vaginal candidiasis

The decision to treat vaginal candidiasis rests on whether the patient has had the symptoms diag-nosed before and whether it is a recurrent prob-lem. If this is the first time the symptoms have appeared or if the woman has had more than two recurrences in the past six months, she should be referred.

The most effective treatment for vulvovaginal candidiasis is one of the imidazole preparations. The choice is between a single-dose oral prep-aration (such as fluconazole) and topical preparations in the form of creams or pessaries (clotrimazole, econazole, miconazole and isoconazole). These are recommended for OTC use only for uncomplicated candidiasis in women who have previously suffered from, and are able to recognise, the condition. Patients may prefer a single-dose treatment either orally or intravaginally.

Imidazole creams may be applied night and morning and can give symptomatic relief where there is extensive vulval or labial irritation. How-ever, an intravaginal preparation or oral dose is necessary to treat the infection, which lies high in the vagina.

Patients with symptoms that have not resolved within seven days should be referred.

Patients should be asked what treatment they have already tried. Creams containing local anaesthetics are widely advertised to the public for this condition but can cause sensitisation and irritation of the perivulval skin. Non-drug rem-edies such as local application of yoghurt or of acidifying agents, such as dilute vinegar, should be discouraged for a few days before and after the use of imidazoles, since the latter are less effec-tive in an acid environment.

Male sexual partners may be asymptomatic carriers of candida, but the value of treating them with antifungal creams is unclear.

Patients should be advised of other measures that can be taken to reduce symptoms. These include avoiding perfumed products, such as soaps and bubble baths, which may exacerbate the skin irritation. Hot baths can cause irritation, as can wearing synthetic underwear, tights and tight fitting trousers.

After defaecation, the anus should be wiped from front to back to prevent transferring infec-tion from the bowel to the vagina.

Imidazoles are inhibitors of the hepatic microsomal metabolism of some drugs. Caution

is therefore advised in patients taking warfarin and it is suggested that the pro-
thrombin ratio (INR, measured routinely in
such patients) be checked within or at the end
of a seven-day treatment period. In theory,
the arrhythmogenic potential of the antihistamines known to cause arrhythmias, i.e.
terfenadine and astemizole, might be enhanced
by both oral and topical imidazoles. Blood
concentrations of theophylline, cyclosporin,
rifampicin and oral sulphonylureas may be
increased by the imidazoles. Except for
cyclosporin, these interactions are unlikely to
be of any clinical significance.

SUMMARY OF CONDITIONS PRODUCING PERIANAL OR PERIVULVAL
PRURITUS

Anal fissure
An anal fissure is a tear in the mucosa of the lower anal canal. It is painful and often associated with
haemorrhoids – **refer**.

Anal fistula
An anal fistula is a deep communicating sinus or channel connecting the anal canal either to the
perineum or to adjacent organs. It causes swelling, pain and pruritus. It is sometimes preceded by an
anorectal abscess – **refer**.

Carcinoma
Cancer of the colon and rectum (see Chapter 8) – **refer**.

Cystitis
Cystitis presents as itching in the urethra, a frequent and an urgent desire to pass urine, and pain on
passing urine. The condition is more common in women than in men. This may be due to organisms being
carried from the perianal area to the urethra, which is relatively short in women so facilitating the passage of bacteria to the bladder. In 50 per cent of cases no bacteria can be isolated from the urine. In
men complaining of these symptoms, referral is necessary to allow investigation, particularly for prostate
and renal causes. Predisposing factors for cystitis include diabetes, trauma during sexual intercourse and
an alteration in the skin environment caused by vaginal deodorants, bubble baths, etc. Treatment with
OTC medicines may be tried for three days in women.

Haemorrhoids
Haemorrhoids are divided into two general types: internal and external. Internal haemorrhoids are
abnormally large or symptomatic dilatations of blood vessels engorged with blood. They are present in
the mucosa of the anal canal, but sometimes may become so swollen with blood that they drop down
outside the anal sphincter (prolapsed haemorrhoids).

External haemorrhoids are of two major types. The first is a swelling in a vessel below the dentate line
(the anorectal line in the anal canal where the skin lining changes to a mucous membrane), which eventually becomes thrombosed, causing the skin to stretch and producing great pain. The second type is a
skin tag – a fibrous appendage covered by skin attached at some point to the circumference of the anus.
They are often formed when a thrombosed external haemorrhoid heals.

Pruritus is a common early symptom of haemorrhoids. There may be bleeding, especially after a bowel

→

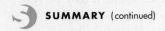

movement. With internal haemorrhoids there is usually no pain unless there is a prolapse, when the patient feels a sensation of something moving down the anal canal, followed by acute pain. External piles are extremely painful – **refer**.

Polyps
Polyps are benign or malignant tumours that can arise anywhere in the large bowel. They are often asymptomatic, but can bleed, cause pain or eventually disturb bowel function to the point of subacute obstruction. Recurrence is common. There is a familial tendency to polyps. If there is a history or family history – **refer**.

Sexually transmitted disease
Those STDs (venereal diseases) that may produce symptoms suggestive of cystitis or candidiasis include the following:

Gonorrhoea
Gonorrhoea is characterised by a urethral discharge in males and a vaginal discharge in females, dysuria and frequency. It usually manifests itself within one week of intercourse – **refer**.

Genital herpes
In genital herpes a vesicular rash affects the tip or shaft of the penis or the labia and vulva. There is local pain, which is aggravated by intercourse, and there may be dysuria – **refer**.

Non-specific urethritis
A variety of causes have been suggested for this condition, including *Chlamydia*, viruses, trichomonas, *Candida* and mixed bacteria. It is seen in men and women and manifests itself as dysuria, frequency and sometimes a slight urethral discharge. It can be passed to babies from the mother during childbirth, causing a potentially blinding eye infection – **refer**.

Genital warts
There are two forms of genital warts: a frond-like growth, which is almost certainly sexually transmitted, and a flat, common skin wart, which is not. Warts affect the labia, vagina and cervix in women and the shaft, glans and particularly the foreskin of men. They may be found around the anus, particularly in homosexual men. They are not serious but are difficult to treat and often recur – **refer**.

Threadworm
Enterobius vermicularis (threadworm) is a small thread-like worm between 3 and 10 mm long. Swallowed ova develop in the gut and infect the large bowel. The female lays eggs outside the anus, usually in warm conditions, such as when the patient is in bed. This causes intense pruritus and sometimes pain, with symptoms being worse at night. Children are particularly susceptible but threadworm spreads in families and at school and all ages can be infested. The condition normally responds to OTC treatment and good hygiene.

Trichomonal vaginitis
Infection by *Trichomonas vaginalis* (trichomoniasis) is rarer than candidal infections. *Trichomonas* is a protozoan. The symptoms of infection with this organism are similar to candidiasis but more severe. The vaginal discharge has an offensive odour and is yellow or green in colour – **refer**.

(continued overleaf)

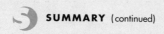

Vaginal candidiasis

Infection with *Candida albicans* (moniliasis, thrush) is probably the most common cause of vaginitis. There is vulvovaginal itching and often an odourless vaginal discharge. Sometimes there is a burning sensation in the vulval area and dysuria. The source of the infection is often the alimentary tract, including the mouth. Infection spreads to the vagina from the anus via the perianal skin. Predisposing factors include pregnancy, diabetes, the use of vaginal deodorants, etc., antibiotics, steroids and possibly oral contraceptives.

Candidiasis may be treated with OTC imidazole preparations if the condition has been previously diagnosed by a doctor. If a patient presents with symptoms suggestive of candidiasis for the first time, she should be referred to confirm the diagnosis. Patients with frequent attacks should be referred to identify the presence of any predisposing factors. Postmenopausal women should also be referred.

Vaginitis caused by other organisms

Chlamydia is a bacterium that may cause cervicitis, vaginitis and salpingitis. Chlamydial infection is sexually transmitted, and is treatable with tetracyclines. *Gardnerella* and *Giardia lamblia* are anaerobic bacteria that occasionally infect the vagina. They are not sensitive to imidazoles and should be suspected if symptoms of vaginitis do not respond to these agents within seven days.

The discharge of bacterial vaginitis is characterised by an offensive smell. It can be distinguished from that of candidiasis in the doctor's surgery or laboratory by a pH of greater than 4.5 (cf. thrush, which has a pH of less than 4.5) and enhancement of the smell by the addition of potassium hydroxide to a sample of the discharge fluid – **refer**.

R   WHEN TO REFER
Perianal and perivulval pruritis

Vaginitis
- Not had before
- Had more than twice in the last six months
- Foul-smelling discharge
- Blood-stained discharge
- Loin pain   Immediate referral if severe
- Abdominal pain   Immediate referral if severe
- Abominal pain and fever and/or vomiting   Immediate
  and diarrhoea
- Pain (other than just soreness) on urination
- Patient is taking immunosuppressants   Immediate
- Patient is diabetic   Immediate
- Pregnancy   Immediate
- Breast feeding
- Age over 60 years
- Age under 16 years
- Failure to improve significantly within
  seven days of OTC treatment
- Ulcers in genital area   Immediate

Threadworm
- Recurrent
- Failure to respond to OTC remedy within a
  few days

Haemorrhoids
- Pain in anal area
- Abdominal pain
- Weight loss
- Age over 40 years and bleeding noted for first
  time
- Going to toilet more frequently
- Failure to respond to OTC products

CASE STUDIES

Case 1

A pleasant man in his late 60s, who is well known to the pharmacist, comes in with a repeat prescription for his usual medication for left ventricular failure and aortic valve disease. He appears unwell, and is obviously anxious. He has just visited the practice nurse for an INR estimation, having had several epistaxes and some spontaneous bruising over the last week or so. The nurse is rightly concerned that his warfarin control, normally stable, needs urgent review, and has questioned him about possible reasons for this, with none discovered.

The pharmacist attempts to reassure him with explanations, but he remains concerned and unconvinced. He fears a serious complication from internal bleeding and thinks he 'may take a chance' and stop the anticoagulation.

Fortunately, at that moment the pharmacist checks the pharmacy records and remembers that the man's wife purchased miconazole cream two weeks before. In a quiet corner they discuss this, and it transpires that she bought it for her husband, who was too embarrassed to reveal a fungal infection in his groin. With permission the doctor is telephoned and reminded of this interaction. The INR is greater than 10, the cream is stopped and control rapidly regained.

Case 2

A well-dressed woman in her late 50s visits her pharmacy and requests a cream for piles. On questioning, she says she has noticed 'something come down' after using the toilet, which is irritant and occasionally streaks the paper with a little fresh blood. She is not keen to talk about it, and a topical application is recommended, with the proviso that she should seek a medical opinion if it persists.

A month later she returns. The medication worked well, there has been no further bleeding but the piles occasionally return. She is convinced they are improving and reluctantly the pharmacist supplies a further tube of cream.

A fortnight later she appears again, this time asking for a laxative. The pharmacist declines, expressing anxiety that the diagnosis must first be confirmed. She is hesitant, her doctor is a young male who helped her through a difficult time around the menopause and with whom she would feel embarrassed. She is eventually persuaded to see the practice nurse (who is female), and returns later to thank the pharmacist. The pharmacist's suspicions were correct – her 'piles' were in fact an early prolapse of the uterus.   The nurse has reassured her that the two are surprisingly often confused, and she is now resigned to await the gynaecology out-patient appointment that has been arranged.

Case 3

A woman in her 30s requests medication for 'worms'. On questioning, threadworms seems the likely diagnosis – two of her three children have perianal itching and one has had small white worms in her stool. When the pharmacist willingly recommends sufficient merbendazole for doses to each of the family members, the youngest of the children, who accompany their mother, breaks into copious tears. Taken aback, the pharmacist reassures the mother and children that there is nothing to fear in this medication. To the pharmacist's surprise, and further alarm, the second child joins the distress of the first. At first reluctant to speak, their mother finally reveals that they are new to this area and have had repeated infections before. Treatment has failed, the children have been banned from school and this is to be their last attempt before the puppy acquired last Christmas must be found a new home, or worse.

Hastily the pharmacist arranges for the pharmacy assistant to occupy the children and takes their

→

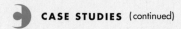

mother to one side. While re-infection from animals is possible, it is unlikely, especially as the dog has been treated and shows no symptoms. He reviews hygiene practice within the family and frequent visitors, and a number of potential human hosts are revealed.

Some time later the family return. The pharmacist, from the back of the shop, is relieved to see them simply buying cosmetics and is even more relieved to observe the presence of a rather attractive mongrel attached to a post outside.

10

Ear disorders

Symptoms in the ear are often associated with upper respiratory tract disorders and are common in children. Symptomatic relief can be obtained in some cases with OTC medicines, but examination of the ear by a doctor is necessary if symptoms persist.

Assessing symptoms

Site or location

Disorders of the ear can be conveniently listed in terms of the site of the lesion (Table 10.1). A diagram of the ear is shown in Figure 10.1.

Table 10.1   Disorders of the ear

Outer ear	Middle ear
Otitis externa:	Otitis media (infection)
(a) dermatitits. (pinna or external ear canal)	Secretory otitis media (glue ear)
(b) infection (external canal)	Trauma and perforation of eardrum
Tumour (pinna)	Otosclerosis
Trauma, e.g. laceration (pinna)	
	Inner ear
Excessive wax (external canal)	Vertigo (including Ménière's disease)
Foreign bodies	Eustachian catarrh or barotrauma
Furuncles (boils)	

Severity

The severity of symptoms in the ear will determine the need for and the urgency of referral. Any severe pain in the middle ear is distressing to the patient and requires an examination with an otoscope by the doctor. If a lesion causing discomfort in the external ear is visible then the pharmacist must make a judgement based on the severity of the symptoms and the possible diagnoses. Thus, dermatitis on the pinna may be itching and uncomfortable, but may be treated with OTC creams in the first instance without the need for referral. On the other hand, a patient with an isolated blister, ulcer or unusual lesion on the pinna, which is growing in size but causing only minimal itch, should be tactfully but firmly referred so that malignancy can be excluded.

Because of its abundant blood supply, trauma to the pinna can result in profuse bleeding. The ear should be compressed with a clean pad and the patient sent to a hospital accident department.

Duration

Acute otitis media generally lasts for less than one week. However, if there is severe pain, referral is necessary before this time so that the ear may be examined to exclude perforation of the eardrum or the development of chronic suppurative otitis media. The latter is more common in adults than in children. Eustachian catarrh, which may accompany the common cold, usually lasts less than one week. Occasionally it may continue and develop into a chronic catarrhal state.

Glue ear (secretory otitis media) may persist

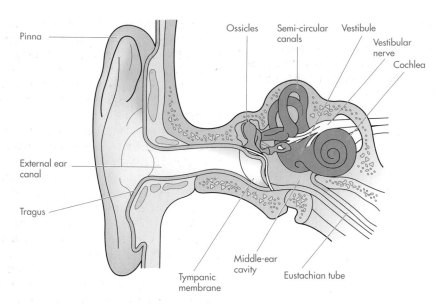

Figure 10.1   Diagram of the ear.

for several weeks or months without being recognised because it is often symptomless until the associated deafness becomes apparent.

Vertigo may occur briefly during an ear infection associated with an upper respiratory tract infection. In such cases, the symptom will resolve in a few days. However, the vertigo associated with Ménière's disease will either persist or recur and become more severe. It will often be accompanied by nausea, vomiting and tinnitus.

Onset

Eustachian catarrh and otitis media may develop during a common cold. Both of these disorders can also be caused by swimming, diving and air travel when pressure differentials between the middle-ear cavity and the outside can suck fluid and micro-organisms from the nasopharynx through the eustachian tube.

Accompanying symptoms

Pain

Pain may be associated with a furuncle (boil) in the external ear canal but otherwise it is not a major feature of otitis externa. Problems caused by earwax do not generally produce pain and it is rarely a major feature of glue ear. Earache is complained of by the majority of patients with otitis media – this is the commonest cause of earache in children. It requires referral for a diagnosis.

Earache may or may not be a feature of eustachian catarrh. It occurs in chronic suppurative otitis media only if the drum perforates. Pain may be experienced during descent in an aircraft (barotrauma), particularly if the sufferer has catarrh.

Earache should generally be regarded as a referrable symptom.

Cold, sore throat

Infection easily passes from the mouth and nasopharynx to the ear via the eustachian tube and ear infections may therefore be the result of bacterial or viral invasion.

Swelling and discharge

Redness, swelling and a discharge are common features of a furuncle in the ear canal but may also reflect an infective dermatitis in the ear canal. A discharge may be seen in both acute and chronic types of otitis media.

Bleeding and bruising

Bleeding in the pinna is often copious and may not respond to the application of pressure. Patients should therefore be referred. In addition, any trauma to the pinna, with or without external bleeding, may result in large haematomas between the skin and the cartilage. These should be assessed by a doctor to determine whether they require draining surgically to prevent fibrous scarring, which can result in the familiar 'cauliflower ear'. Any blood discharged into the ear canal requires a medical opinion to exclude perforation of the eardrum if the bleeding does not appear to arise from the ear canal.

Itching

Itching or irritation of the ear canal or pinna usually represents a form of dermatitis, which can be treated with OTC topical preparations. It may sometimes be caused by the presence of a discharge in the canal.

Deafness

Deafness can be caused by obstruction in the external ear canal, inflammation in the middle or inner ear or a disturbance of the auditory nerve. It is therefore to be expected when the ear canal is blocked by wax, debris or a discharge (as from an infection), and in otitis media (chronic and acute), eustachian catarrh and barotrauma. In glue ear the onset of deafness is insidious and may only be recognised when a child is observed to be failing at school because he/she cannot hear properly. Deafness with no apparent cause in young adults may be due to otosclerosis (see p 109) or may be industrial deafness, a permanent result of long-term unprotected exposure to high levels of noise, mostly from machinery.

Deafness can be tested with a tuning fork to determine whether it is conductive or perceptive. Conductive deafness is caused by failure of conduction of sound waves. Normally, sound waves enter the ear canal and cause the eardrum to vibrate, which then moves the chain of ossicles to transmit the vibrations to the cochlea in the inner ear. Perceptive deafness is failure of the system beyond this point, such as the cochlea failing to transmit the vibrations and stimulate the auditory nerve, or the nerve itself failing to transmit impulses so that the sound can be appreciated in the brain.

Red eardrum

Using an otoscope, many ear conditions can be differentiated by the state of the tympanic membrane (eardrum). It appears normal in otitis externa, is often normal in glue ear, but is red in otitis media or following trauma. This is important, since the instillation of ear drops is contraindicated when the drum is perforated. Often the drum cannot be seen during examination with an otoscope because of occlusion by a discharge or wax.

Fever and malaise

Otitis externa does not usually produce any signs of systemic disturbance, even in the case of a furuncle in the ear canal, unless the infection is severe. Fever is generally a sign of infection and is common in children with otitis media; it is often accompanied by vomiting. It is also a common sign of teething in babies with earache.

Something in the ear

Although patients may describe occlusion of the ear canal and the associated deafness as a feeling of something in the ear, it should be remembered that foreign bodies can also represent real rather than imaginary objects. They can cause anxiety and, in the case of live insects, acute pain and appalling irritation as they struggle and flap their wings. Insects can be dealt with in the first instance by the pharmacist (see Management). Foreign bodies may sometimes be removed, depending on what the object is and its accessibility.

Neck stiffness

Neck stiffness associated with symptoms in the ear requires referral to exclude the rare cases of an abscess in the mastoid air cells, or thrombosis of the adjacent cavernous venous sinus, the associated inflammation spreading to involve the meninges or even the brain.

Tinnitus

Tinnitus is the complaint of an extraneous noise arising in the ear or anywhere in the head. It is usually described as ringing, buzzing, hissing or even pulsating. It may be a symptom of any disorder of the ear. It can be an accompaniment of senile deafness, otosclerosis, industrial deafness, Ménière's disease or drug toxicity [e.g. high-dose aspirin, frusemide (furosemide), gentamicin].

Vertigo

Disturbances of the inner ear may cause vertigo, the most important causes being Ménière's disease, vestibular neuronitis and positional (postural) vertigo. Vertigo is best described as a sensation of the room spinning around the sufferer. It should be distinguished from unsteadiness on the feet (as occurs, for example, in muscle weakness or Parkinson's disease) or lightheadedness (a feeling of dizziness, as in postural hypotension, which may be associated with some drugs, particularly antihypertensive drugs in elderly patients). Vertigo is a referrable symptom if it occurs at some time of the day for more than a few days.

Nausea and vomiting

Nausea and vomiting in association with vertigo, tinnitus and eventual deafness is seen typically in Ménière's disease but may also reflect other disorders in the internal ear.

Incidence and recurrence

As might be expected, infections of the middle ear (otitis media) are more common in winter because of the association with upper respiratory infections. In the summer, such infections may result from swimming, diving and air travel. Symptoms may not become significant until several days after acquiring the infection and patients should be questioned about their activities, especially after a holiday.

Glue ear can develop into a chronic condition but it may be difficult to identify until deafness becomes apparent.

Otitis externa can also develop into a chronic condition that is symptomatic from time to time.

Trigger factors

Recurrent episodes of otitis media may be associated with swimming and water sports. In children, frequent upper respiratory infections and attacks of otitis media may be associated with the development of a persistent catarrhal problem. Repeated barotrauma in frequent air travellers can have the same effect.

Patients who have an inflammatory lesion, such as a furuncle in the ear canal, will complain that it is painful when the pinna is pulled upwards and back (as when an observer attempts to examine the ear) or when the tragus is pressed.

Patients with positional vertigo will often have momentary vertigo when getting out of bed.

Management

Problems of the external ear

Dry skin on the pinna can be treated with an emollient such as aqueous cream, emulsifying ointment or a similar proprietary preparation. If the skin of the external ear canal is affected, olive oil may be more convenient to use. If there is a contact dermatitis caused by sensitivity to earrings, patients should be encouraged to wear nickel-free earrings or to use a proprietary clear lacquer to coat the earrings so that the nickel is not in contact with the skin. Topical hydrocortisone should also be used in such a case of contact dermatitis, provided that the pharmacist is confident there is no infection present.

Aluminium acetate solution may be a useful astringent for itching otitis externa and can be used when there is a wet dermatitis either on the pinna or in the ear canal.

If an infection is suspected or the lesion is not showing signs of improvement after seven days, the patient should be advised to see a doctor to evaluate the need for antibiotics.

Many cases of otitis externa affecting the external ear canal are aggravated by water and by scratching. These factors, and poor cleaning of the ear, will predispose to infection. The patient should be advised either to avoid swimming or at least to use earplugs when doing so, to dry the ears gently but thoroughly and to perform an aural toilet before instilling drops into the ear canal. The removal of debris from the ear canal and the maintenance of a clean, dry environment will deter invasion by pathogenic organisms. Cleaning should be done with cotton wool buds, which should be used once and then disposed of. The cotton wool should be gently rotated along the entire length of the canal.

Although it is necessary to keep the canal dry, it should not be occluded with a plug (except when swimming) if there is any exudate, as this will only serve to keep the exudate inside and provoke further irritation. The use of an appropriate proprietary preparation or aluminium acetate solution should assist in drying up excess moisture and such a preparation can be used prophylactically.

Adults should be told not to poke hard objects, such as hair grips or match sticks, down the ear canal as they may scratch the canal and promote infection, and there is also a small risk that the eardrum may become perforated.

Fretful children who writhe are at risk of damage to the ear during cleaning. They are best dealt with by sitting the child sideways on the parent's lap while another person performs the cleaning procedure. One parental arm can be placed around the child's shoulders and the other around its head, holding this against the chest.

Furuncles in the ear canal are difficult to treat but some relief can be obtained by the application of a hot flannel and oral analgesics.

Cerumenolytics

Water- or oil-based ear drops can be used to dissolve excess wax. They are not always successful and take several days to produce their effect. However, they do facilitate syringing, which may have to be resorted to by the doctor or practice nurse if the drops alone are not effective within one week. Problems may arise if drops are instilled into an ear with a perforated drum since this may cause irritation or pain and perhaps infection of the middle ear.

It is often impossible to visualise the eardrum using an otoscope when there is a large amount of wax in the canal and the doctor then has to rely on taking a brief history to assess the likelihood of a perforated drum. This can be done by a pharmacist by asking if the patient has had a recent ear infection or whether there has been a history of perforation or a chronically discharging ear. Perforation may have occurred recently without being diagnosed by a doctor and thus the patient should be asked about any discomfort or pain, especially after diving or any other water sports or air travel. If any of these questions are answered in the affirmative, the patient should be referred. Similarly, if patients experience pain when instilling ear drops, they should be referred.

Some cerumenolytics will sometimes cause earwax to swell at first and patients should be warned that deafness may be worsened initially.

Several proprietary drops contain wetting agents, such as docusate, which may be helpful. On the other hand, some contain potential irritants such as chlorobutanol and paradichlorobenzene. Their use is contraindicated in the presence of otitis externa and patients should be warned to discontinue usage if any discomfort is felt.

It is difficult to assess the comparative efficacy of cerumenolytics from the literature and many doctors hold the view that simple generic preparations such as olive oil or sodium bicarbonate drops are satisfactory.

Removal of foreign bodies

Removal of foreign bodies from the ear (usually of a child) is best left to an expert unless the object is easy to grip with either fingernails or forceps and the pharmacist is particularly dextrous. This is because the eardrum is easily damaged or the object can be inadvertently pushed further into the canal. If a live insect is in the ear canal, a few drops of olive oil should cause a speedy demise of the intruder and the patient should then be referred to the doctor to have the remains syringed out. If the insect has stung the patient, producing oedema and occlusion of the ear canal, referral to an accident and emergency department is necessary.

Eustachian catarrh

Measures can be taken to prevent and treat eustachian catarrh or barotrauma. The aim is to force air up the eustachian tube to allow ventilation of the middle ear. Sucking sweets, swallowing, using earplugs or Valsalva's manoeuvre are all useful. Valsalva's manoeuvre involves pinching the nose, closing the mouth and then trying to breathe out.

Both eustachian catarrh and barotrauma can be treated with oral or topical nasal decongestants. If drops are used, the patient should be told to lie down with the head extended and to remain in that position for five minutes after nasal instillation so that the drops will travel down and backwards to the postnasal space and the oropharynx, where the entrance to the eustachian tube lies. Oral analgesics and local warming may also give symptomatic relief in the condition.

Middle-ear conditions

Otitis media is usually treated primarily with antibiotics, but these may be supported with oral analgesics and nasal vasoconstrictor drops, and the pharmacist may wish to advise on their choice and usage. However, the benefits of antibiotic treatment in acute otitis media are controversial and in some cases doctors will prefer not to prescribe them.

Ear drops containing analgesics are unlikely to have any advantage over oral analgesics.

If the eardrum is perforated, swimming is best avoided or earplugs should be used.

Episodes of acute otitis media accompanying chronic glue ear will be similarly treated with antibiotics and decongestants. In children, radical treatment of glue ear takes the form of myringotomy (incision of the eardrum) and drainage of the effusion. The cavity is then kept dry by inserting a grommet in the hole in the drum and this remains in place for several months.

SUMMARY OF CONDITIONS PRODUCING EAR DISORDERS

Eustachian catarrh and barotrauma

Blockage of the eustachian tube causes air to be absorbed from the middle ear. This results in the eardrum being drawn in. The main symptom is transient pain and deafness, which usually resolves itself in a few days. It may follow a respiratory infection [usually in children (eustachian catarrh)] or mechanical pressure factors such as diving and rapid descent in an aircraft [often in adults (barotrauma)]. In such circumstances, the air pressure outside the middle ear is greater than that inside and the air is sucked up the eustachian tube, which then occludes. If deafness persists for two or three days – **refer**.

Furuncles

A furuncle (boil) in the external ear canal is painful and if the ear canal is obstructed it may cause deafness. There may be a discharge. When the boil bursts, the pain will subside. It may respond to OTC analgesics, but if the pain is severe or there is deafness – **refer**.

Ménière's disease

The symptoms of Ménière's disease are caused by increased pressure of the fluid in the labyrinth (the organ of balance). The cause of the condition is not understood. The patient suffers attacks of vertigo which increase in severity and frequency. There is also nausea and vomiting, tinnitus and a perceptive deafness – **refer**.

Otitis externa

Otitis externa is inflammation of the skin of the pinna or external ear canal. It may be infective or reactive. The infective type is caused by bacteria, viruses or fungi. An exudate is discharged, which may block the external ear canal. In the reactive type, the condition is seen as a form of dermatitis, which may be atopic or a contact dermatitis, most commonly related to earrings. Often a dermatitis will become infected and the two types of otitis externa will coexist. The ear canal will be sore and itching in either type, but in the purely reactive type the skin will usually be dry, red and sometimes scaly. This condition may be treated with OTC preparations. If infective – **refer**.

Otitis media

Acute otitis media is a bacterial or viral infection of the middle ear. *Streptococcus* is the main bacterial pathogen. It often follows an upper respiratory infection. Children are most commonly affected. It causes pain, discharge and often fever. Perforation of the eardrum may occur, in which case the release of pressure on the drum relieves the pain, but the discharge will persist. Chronic suppurative otitis media usually follows perforation of the drum in acute otitis media, resulting in superinfection with other bacteria. Antibacterial treatment usually resolves or, if given early enough, prevents the condition – **refer**.

Otosclerosis

Otosclerosis is a cause of deafness in which there is deposition of new bone around one of the ossicles (the stapes) in the inner ear, preventing conduction of the vibrations of the eardrum to the cochlea. It usually begins unilaterally, mainly in young adults, and it may be some years from its onset before deafness is noted. Tinnitus is sometimes present. There is often a family history – **refer**.

(continued overleaf)

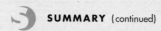 **SUMMARY** (continued)

Secretory otitis media
This condition, also known as glue ear or chronic or serous catarrhal otitis media, is a condition mainly of children. The middle-ear space becomes full of a sticky effusion (hence the term 'glue ear'), the escape of which is impeded by some obstruction or defect in the eustachian tube. It is symptomless, apart from impairment of hearing, which is often undiagnosed for some time but may be suspected following frequent and recurrent middle-ear infections – **refer**.

Tumours
Skin cancers may develop on the pinna of the ear, and are sometimes related to exposure to the sun. Any lesion that persists or causes discomfort should be treated with suspicion. Basal cell carcinomas (rodent ulcers) appear as a central ulcer surrounded by a raised, rolled edge. An epithelioma usually appears as a smooth rounded tumour, but may develop an uneven 'warty' surface. Melanomas are almost always pigmented and may be new occurrences or may be suspected in an existing mole that undergoes any change, especially if it is traumatised by sun damage, spectacle frames or scratching – **refer**.

Vestibular neuronitis
Also known as epidemic vertigo, this condition presents as an attack of vertigo associated with a febrile upper respiratory infection. It is probably a viral invasion of the ear and usually resolves within a few days with bedrest. Hearing is not affected, in comparison with Ménière's disease – **refer**.

Wax
Wax is produced in every ear in varying amounts. If it accumulates in the ear canal, it may dry and harden to form a solid plug, which can obstruct the ear canal. This prevents transmission of sound waves to the eardrum and results in hearing impairment. It may be treated in the first instance with OTC ear drops, but if persistent – **refer**.

WHEN TO REFER
Ear disorders

- Pain
- Deafness
- History or suspicion of a perforated eardrum
- Abnormal lesion/blister/ulcer
- Persistent vertigo
- Tinnitus
- Persistent wax
- Eustachian catarrh before air travel

Ear canal
- Discharge
- Foreign body
- Dermatitis/erythema/irritation that contraindicates the use of ear drops

Pinna
- Profuse bleeding/bruising (refer to accident and emergency department)
- Trauma
- Swelling
- Redness (unless due to allergic eczema)

Accompanying symptoms
- Nausea and vomiting
- Neck stiffness

CASE STUDIES

Case 1

A young woman with a child of about 8 years old presents the pharmacist with a prescription for a small quantity of paediatric paracetamol. As she waits for this to be made up it becomes apparent that she is restless and increasingly agitated. When it is finally ready she snaps, 'Will this do any good?' The pharmacist therefore takes a brief history. The child has just visited the doctor with an episode of earache. It started two nights before, and the pain is less severe now than at first, but the mother is understandably anxious that it does not worsen again, and that no damage to the ear results. The pharmacist remembers previous prescriptions, often for antibiotics. There is a history of recurrent infection. The most recent was only a few weeks before.

The pharmacist attempts to explain. She is quite right to be concerned, and to seek assessment when her child has earache. Some such cases will be caused by bacterial infection and will require antibiotics to resolve them and help prevent middle-ear damage. However, in some instances, such as now, when the condition appears to be improving, it may be better not to treat in this way. The problem may well have been a catarrhal obstruction rather than an infection. With a history of frequent infections, withholding antibiotics, when it is feasible, helps prevent development of resistance so that they can be relied on to be effective in cases when they are used. Finally, some doctors believe repeated antibiotic use may predispose the development of catarrhal states such as glue ear.

The woman understands this explanation, but remembers two nights ago and the lost sleep for both of them. The pharmacist attempts to meet her halfway by recommending decongestant nasal drops, which when used correctly work quickly and can be useful in an emergency. If the pain does persist, the pharmacist says she should certainly have the situation reviewed as advised.

The woman leaves in a calmer state than when she entered, and the pharmacist reflects on how often it is necessary to offer a medicine to maintain confidence as much as to treat.

Case 2

A smartly dressed young woman in her mid 20s comes into the pharmacy. It is Friday, she cannot see her doctor until next week and she is keen to speak to the pharmacist. She is an air stewardess and is due to fly again over the weekend. She has had a cold or similar catarrhal condition and feels her ears are blocked. She has had pain once before on descent and fears a tympanic membrane rupture. Could the pharmacist give her some antibiotics and square it with the doctor on Monday?

Antibiotics, the pharmacist explains, will not help a eustachian blockage. In a modern pressurised aircraft the risk of perforation is very low, but the chance of pain from barotrauma is somewhat more likely. In any case, the woman would obviously be anxious and possibly unable to continue her work. Would it not be more sensible, suggests the pharmacist, to miss this next shift and allow the condition to settle? The woman is reluctant to do this, having taken time off before and fearing for her job. A second missed shift could mean a referral to the company doctor and the prospect of grounding. The pharmacist sympathises, but points out that the airline would not take such action unless there was a reason. Perhaps a compromise is called for. The pharmacist suggests using a decongestant immediately, which if successful would allow her to fly. If this does not work, then a trip to the doctor for otoscopic examination and diagnosis can be made. This, after all, is a common problem and one that can usually be resolved.

→

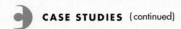 **CASE STUDIES** (continued)

Case 3

A middle-aged man asks for the pharmacist's advice. Over the last few weeks he has become progressively deaf, more on one side than on the other, and has the feeling his ears are full up. He has had problems with wax accumulation before and this seems likely to be the problem now.

The pharmacist checks the man's history. The man has never had a perforated drum, and has had his ears syringed in the past. There is no history of middle-ear infection since the last syringing, about two years ago. The man asks for cerumenolytic drops, which the pharmacist is happy to provide.

The man also asks whether it will be necessary to make an appointment with the practice nurse for ear syringing or whether the drops will be sufficient. The pharmacist replies that to have enough wax to notice a marked hearing loss implies a lot of debris and while the drops will loosen it, they may not remove it completely. The pharmacist suggests making an appointment, which will take a few days anyway, but being prepared to cancel it should a reasonable quantity of wax be discharged and the symptoms resolve. In any case, it would be wise to have the nurse at least check his ears to be sure.

Shoulder

The most common disorder affecting the shoulder joint, apart from trauma, is capsulitis (rotator cuff syndrome). This may be caused by overuse or unaccustomed movement resulting in inflammation in the ring of tendons attached to the shoulder muscles. Movement is restricted in one or all directions.

A common variant is the supraspinatus syndrome. The supraspinatus muscle, which lies on the upper border of the spine of the scapula, is responsible for abduction (raising) of the arm at the shoulder joint. In this syndrome the shoulder is particularly painful when the patient is asked to raise his arm laterally from the body. Palpation at the outermost point of the shoulder, just behind the lateral tip of the clavicle, will reveal an acutely tender supraspinatus tendon, confirming the diagnosis. In the more widespread rotator cuff syndrome, the tenderness is slightly lower, around the neck of the humerus, and extends further.

After a painful disorder of the shoulder has apparently healed, it may become apparent some time afterwards that the arm cannot be raised above the head or behind the back. This is often due to scarring or fibrosis of the muscles, tendons and ligaments around the shoulder joint, which can occur to such an extent that the syndrome known as frozen shoulder develops, often with some degree of irreversibility.

Back

Thoracic spine

Thoracic spinal pain is uncommon and should be referred unless some obvious trivial cause can be found.

Pain arising in the intercostal muscles (between the ribs) may be due to a muscle strain, but must be distinguished from the pain of a myocardial infarction, pulmonary embolus or pleurisy.

Pain arising after straining, while lifting a heavy object or coughing, may be due to a muscle strain or tear, or to a prolapsed (slipped) disc, which will cause a ligament to be stretched

and muscles to go into spasm. Such musculoskeletal damage must be differentiated from other serious causes of pain. Chest pain due to angina will usually disappear after resting or, if there is a history and the patient has medication, after glyceryl trinitrate. The pain of myocardial infarction lasts longer than 30 minutes and the patient will often be anxious, cyanosed and sweating, and, in most cases, will be obviously ill. A muscle strain or tear will cause a sharp pain in a small, defined area and will be exacerbated by coughing or deep inspiration. This is also the case with pleurisy or a pulmonary embolus, although in severe cases of these disorders the pain may be present continuously with abnormal breathing.

If these latter diagnoses cannot be excluded, the patient should be referred.

Lumbar spine

Low back pain, often referred to as lumbago, may be mild or severe. In both types there will often be a strain of the spinal muscles and ligaments. In the more severe type the patient should be encouraged to rest to see if the symptoms resolve. Sometimes the cause can be a prolapsed intervertebral disc and, in such cases, harm can be done by the patient 'soldiering on'.

The pain of a prolapsed disc is constant but is exacerbated by movement. The patient will hold him- or herself rigid to avoid movement. The patient's gait will be stiff and awkward.

A prolapsed disc (see Figure 11.1) will often impinge on the roots of nerves originating from the spinal cord, the most commonly affected being the sciatic nerve. In such cases, the pressure on the nerve root will cause pain in the area supplied by the nerve. This is called sciatica. The pain may be intense and burning, radiating from the back to the buttock and the back of the leg and sometimes to the front of the thigh. It may spread to below the knee. The patient with sciatica will limp and will be unable to flex the hip very far, making climbing stairs or sitting down uncomfortable. If a prolapsed disc is suspected, the patient should be referred.

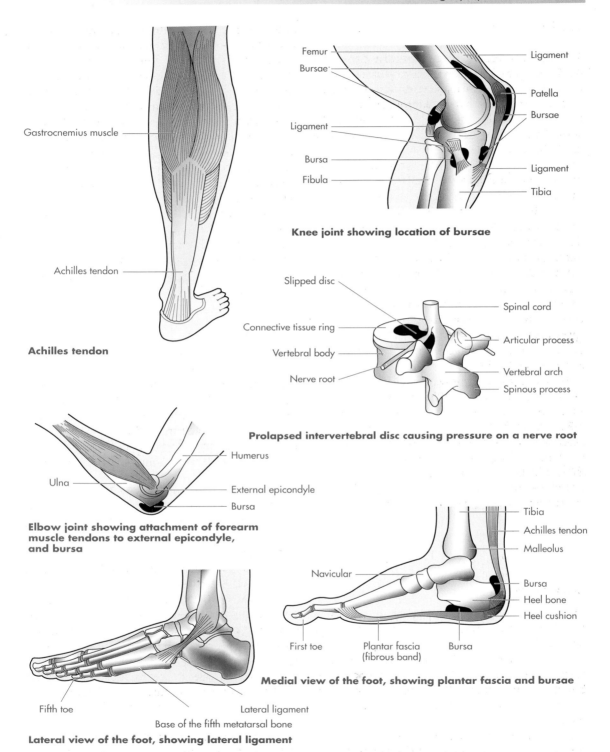

Gastrocnemius muscle

Achilles tendon

Achilles tendon

Femur
Bursae
Ligament
Bursa
Fibula

Ligament
Patella
Bursae
Ligament
Tibia

Knee joint showing location of bursae

Slipped disc
Connective tissue ring
Vertebral body
Nerve root

Spinal cord
Articular process
Vertebral arch
Spinous process

Prolapsed intervertebral disc causing pressure on a nerve root

Humerus
Ulna
External epicondyle
Bursa

Elbow joint showing attachment of forearm muscle tendons to external epicondyle, and bursa

Tibia
Achilles tendon
Malleolus
Navicular
Bursa
Heel bone
Heel cushion
First toe
Plantar fascia (fibrous band)
Bursa

Medial view of the foot, showing plantar fascia and bursae

Fifth toe
Lateral ligament
Base of the fifth metatarsal bone

Lateral view of the foot, showing lateral ligament

Figure 11.1 Diagrams showing parts of joints.

Acute soft tissue lumbago (strain of a ligament or muscle) can often be related to an event such as lifting or twisting. The pain may be experienced diffusely across both sides of the back at the level of the sacrum or linearly and to one side in the vertically running spinal muscles. There is often no pain at rest or on slow movement. Chronic lumbago is common but very difficult to treat. Any history of a sporting, car or industrial injury, previous slipped disc or arthritis will require medical referral.

It should always be borne in mind that diseases of various organs can cause backache. Inquiry should be made to exclude discomfort on micturition or colicky abdominal pain which may indicate a urinary tract infection or renal colic. In women, any cyclical low back pain should be viewed with caution, particularly if it occurs in the middle or second half of the menstrual cycle, as this warrants consideration of a non-musculoskeletal cause. Inquiry about any menstrual irregularity or abdominal pain should be made but even in the absence of these symptoms recurrent cyclical pain requires referral.

Any change in bowel habit or any weight loss should be viewed with suspicion since it may reflect a disorder in the large bowel, which lies close to the sacral area of the lower back.

Persistent unexplained lumbar pain in middle age and beyond could indicate a malignant secondary tumour and must be investigated.

Coccygitis

Coccygitis produces a pain in the coccyx (tailbone) and is often caused by a fall on to a hard surface. The coccyx will be tender to the touch and painful, especially when sitting down. It takes a few weeks to heal.

Elbow

Various types of injury to the elbow or overuse of the muscles associated with it, which control wrist and finger movements, may be seen.

Location

Pain and tenderness to the touch around the small bony protuberance on the outer side of the elbow is characteristic of tennis elbow (see Figure 11.1). Similarly, pain and tenderness around the bony protuberance on the inner side of the elbow is known as golfer's elbow. These protuberances are the epicondyles and the bony pains of tennis and golfer's elbow are known as lateral and medial epicondylitis, respectively.

Pain and tenderness over the tip of the elbow (the olecranon) is popularly known as student's elbow.

Duration

The symptoms of any of these syndromes will last a varying amount of time depending on the severity of the problem. Symptoms that persist for more than one or two weeks should be referred if they are particularly troublesome.

Onset, spread of symptoms and aggravating factors

Despite their popular names, it is not only golfers, tennis players and students who suffer these symptoms.

Student's elbow can be caused either by inflammation of, or bleeding into, a bursa at the tip of the elbow. It is fairly easy to diagnose without inquiry about its onset, although there may be a classic history of a blow to, or fall on to, the elbow, repeated flexing of the elbow or persistent leaning on the elbow in such recreational pursuits as drinking or rifle shooting. Pain will be felt at rest and on movement of the elbow and there may be swelling and redness. The swelling can extend to the forearm.

Tennis and golfer's elbow can be traced to overuse or unaccustomed movement, such as curling of the wrist as in powerful gripping and pulling actions, which strains the tendons of the forearm muscles attached to the outer (tennis) or the inner (golfer's) epicondyles at the elbow. The resulting stress on the elbow produces pain in both the elbow and the forearm muscles and a weakness of the wrist. Flexing the hand downwards at the wrist joint will cause pain in golfer's

Chondro = related to cartilage.
malacia = softening

elbow and bending the hand back at the wrist will cause pain in tennis elbow.

Pain may spread to the inner aspects of the forearm in golfer's elbow and to the outer forearm in tennis elbow.

Forearm, wrist and hand

Pain in the forearm, wrist and hand can be caused by entrapment of nerves. The most common presentations of this type of disorder are tenosynovitis and carpal tunnel syndrome. Both conditions can produce pain and tenderness over the flexor surface of the forearm. If the pain is also felt in the palm of the hand, fingers and wrist, it suggests carpal tunnel involvement.

Treatment of mild cases of both conditions is similar, so that a definitive diagnosis is not important, but if suspected the patient should be referred.

Upper leg

Pain in the upper leg, apart from sciatica (see above), will probably be caused either by a strain or rupture of the thigh muscles or by cramp-like stiffness after unaccustomed exercise.

Onset and accompanying symptoms

A sudden stabbing pain in the anterior thigh after a rapid contraction of the muscles, e.g. when an athlete or sports player makes a forceful sudden movement, will most likely be due to a rupture of the quadriceps muscle. Pain at the back of the thigh will be caused by similar damage to the hamstring muscle. There will be tenderness and often bruising and swelling.

Knee

In young patients, traumatic injuries to the knee are relatively common, whereas in older patients, painful knees are often caused by osteoarthritis.

A swelling or lump on the back of the knee is likely to be due to a distended bursa, a condition known as Baker's cyst. The swelling is usually at least the size of a golf ball and is caused by leakage from an inflamed knee joint into the bursa at the back of the knee (see Figure 11.1).

Pain over the knee with a swelling of the joint may be caused by pre-patellar bursitis, popularly known as housemaid's knee.

Onset

Certain events, usually in sport, such as twisting, turning or a lateral impact as in soccer when two players kick the ball at the same time with the inside of their feet, may precipitate injuries to the joint capsule or its associated ligaments and the cartilages inside the joint itself.

Pain in the knee joint that is noticed for the first time when walking up and down hills or stairs (and is worse walking down) may be due to chondromalacia patellae. This condition involves thickening of the cartilage lining the kneecap, and is caused by overuse. A similar condition in young people causing pain and inflammation just below the kneecap, particularly on exercise, is called Osgood–Schlatter's disease.

Ankle

An ankle sprain is the most common soft tissue limb injury and commonly presents with a history of excessive movement on the joint.

The lateral ligament attaches the fibula (the thinner, outer bone in the lower leg) to the heel and foot bones on the outer side of the ankle joint (see Figure 11.1). The lateral ligament is weaker than the broader medial ligament, which attaches the tibia bone to the heel bone on the inner aspect of the ankle. Sprains are caused by an inversion injury to the lateral ligament. Swelling over the lateral ligament below the ankle is less significant than swelling over the lateral ankle joint.

There is usually swelling and tenderness around the front and side of the ankle. It is sometimes difficult to distinguish between a fracture and a ligament injury (sprain) and if in doubt patients should be persuaded to have an X-ray. However, the following guidelines to referral will be helpful:

- Refer if there is bone tenderness of either the bony protuberance of the ankle (malleolus), the navicular bone in the foot just below the ankle joint on the instep or the base of the fifth metatarsal bone on the outer edge of the foot (see Figure 11.1)
- Refer if the patient cannot weight bear for at least four steps
- Refer if there is pain at rest.

Lower leg

Pain in the front middle part of the shin bone can be caused by an overuse injury. Other problems in the lower leg include sprained ankle, ruptured Achilles tendon (see Figure 11.1) and cramp in the calf.

Ruptures of muscles in the calf and of the Achilles tendon are common in sport injuries but can also occur in non-sporting, day-to-day situations.

A sudden pain in the calf, as though hit on the back of the leg, with tenderness and difficulty in contracting the calf muscles, may be due to rupture of the calf muscles (the gastrocnemius and soleus).

A ruptured Achilles tendon is intensely painful over the Achilles area, which lies above the heel and below the calf muscles. There is often a classic history of a blow or a kick on the back of the leg and the tendon can sometimes be heard to snap. Medical referral is necessary.

Where the tendon is totally ruptured, the patient will not be able to walk on the affected foot. Indentation may be noted in the tendon at the sight of injury. In milder cases, such as partial rupture or tendinitis (inflammation of the tendon), there will be difficulty in standing on tiptoe. Even mild cases, where the injury to the tendon is slight, must be referred for proper examination and advice. The condition could otherwise result in scarring of the tendon, which is liable to become chronically inflamed.

Muscle cramps are common in the calf muscles, not only during strenuous exercise but also at rest. They are experienced particularly by the elderly.

Foot

A painful heel may be the result of bursitis. Pain at the back of the heel may be due to inflammation of a deep bursa lying between the heelbone and the attachment of the Achilles tendon or a superficial tendon located under the skin (see Figure 11.1). There may be redness and swelling and it may become difficult to wear normal shoes.

In children up to the age of 18 years, fragmentation of the Achilles tendon attachment to the heelbone can occur, causing pain at the back of the heel during and for some time after walking or running.

Pain under the heel may be due to rupture of connective tissue below the heel. In such cases, the heelbone becomes less firmly held and squeezes the cushion of fat normally beneath it to the side. This causes pressure on the skin, resulting in pain. There is also a bursa between the heelbone and the fat cushion which may become inflamed.

Pain under the heel, often with pain in the sole, is commonly due to plantar fasciitis. This occurs where the arch ligaments (running under the foot from the toes to the heel) are stretched or damaged. The pain is relieved on rest, and is worse when on tiptoe or walking on the heels. There may be stiffness, particularly in the mornings.

Special considerations

Pregnancy

Because of the extra load placed on the skeleton by the growing foetus, lumbago is a common problem in pregnancy. Patients should be reassured, but if the pain is unbearable they are best referred. Musculoskeletal problems in pregnancy are commonly mechanical, the growing load being asymetrically distributed. They may also be metabolic or related to pressure effects on the pelvic floor, blood vessels or other organs. Exercising opposing muscle groups to stretch the affected part may relieve the pain and spasm. If the condition is persistently troublesome, referral can be made.

Management

Treatment of acute soft tissue injury where there may be bleeding, for example in sports injuries and acute bursitis, should be immediate. The aim is to stop the bleeding, swelling, pain and tenderness. Bleeding can also delay healing, make infection more likely and distort scar tissue formation, producing a cosmetically poor result and possibly interfering with function.

The well-known mnemonic RICE comes into play. It represents Rest, Ice, Compression and Elevation.

Rest and elevation

Rest allows immobilisation, which enhances healing and reduces blood flow to the affected tissue. Rest should ideally be for 24 to 48 hours, but this is often difficult to achieve. Elevation of the affected part also reduces blood flow and leakage of fluid into the extracellular spaces.

Cooling

Ice packs are used to reduce blood flow to injured tissue and thus reduce bleeding and swelling. Cooling also has an analgesic effect. Ice packs should be separated from the skin by a thin towel or a handkerchief to prevent skin damage. To be effective, cooling should be continued for at least 30 minutes in, for example, a knee or ankle injury, and longer if the injury is particularly severe or when deep large muscles are involved, as in the thigh. One disadvantage of cooling is that it may encourage someone to begin exercising the affected part of the body too soon after an injury, thus causing more bleeding and delaying healing.

Cooling aerosol sprays can exert an analgesic effect if a bone that lies close to the skin, such as the ankle or shin, has been knocked. Sprays only penetrate into the skin layer. They can, however, cause injury to the skin if they are not used carefully and should not be applied to broken skin. Their brief and superficial action

means that when cooling has ceased, the blood flow increases and any beneficial effect may be lost.

Compression

Compression of an acute injury allows haemostasis to occur, and thereby reduces swelling. A supportive bandage, such as a crepe bandage or an elastocrepe, can be applied. Elasticated sports supports designed for specific areas are available.

Heat

Heat or massage will have the opposite effect on blood flow to that of cooling. It should therefore not be used until about 48 hours after an acute injury, i.e. when the risk of bleeding has disappeared. Heat offers relief from pain arising from inflammation or overuse.

As well as being of value in trauma heat is also effective in chronic joint pain such as rheumatoid arthritis and osteoarthritis, wry neck, backache and deep muscle pain. Heat decreases joint stiffness and relieves muscle spasm. It increases the elasticity and plasticity of collagen fibres in tissues such as tendons, preventing them from becoming stiff, and also aids gentle exercise in the rehabilitation phase.

Heat may be generated in the form of topical medication (see below), infra-red lamps, heating pads, hot baths or by ultrasound treatment, which is used by physiotherapists. Heat retainers commonly worn by sportsmen are supports made of synthetic material which generate and retain heat as well as giving useful support and improving the mobility of joints and limbs.

Heat is useful in preventing injury, which explains the importance of warm-up exercises, especially in cold weather.

Topical medication

Topical medication applied to aches and pains is a traditional remedy and is generally effective. Most preparations cause vasodilatation and produce a sensation of warmth. They encourage healing and also provide analgesia. They are useful as a preventative and rehabilitative measure, but should not be used in the acute stage of injury, when there is a risk of bleeding.

The traditional constituent of embrocations and liniments is methyl salicylate, present in many proprietary balms, liniments and balsams. The concentration varies between different products and the pharmacist should be aware of a possible difference in potencies because of this. Branded products also often include turpentine oil and a variety of salicylates and nicotinates. The efficacy of most topical medications is enhanced by massage during application, which will itself induce vasodilatation.

Topical preparations of the NSAIDs ibuprofen, ketoprofen, diclofenac, felbinac and piroxicam are useful analgesic and anti-inflammatory agents. There has been considerable controversy about the efficacy of topical NSAIDs, but they do provide symptomatic relief in some patients and can be used for muscular aches, sprains and strains, and rheumatoid symptoms. They can be used immediately after acute injury.

Oral analgesics

Simple analgesics such as paracetamol and the NSAIDs aspirin and ibuprofen can give effective relief of musculoskeletal pain when used either alone or in conjunction with other treatments. They may be helpful in acute injury as well as more chronic conditions such as torticollis, sterno-costal joint strain, frozen shoulder, carpal tunnel syndrome, back pain and coccygitis. Care should be taken to inquire about any relative contraindications to NSAIDs, such as a history of peptic ulcer or upper gastrointestinal disorders and asthma.

Patients with chronic pain or stiffness should be referred for assessment. In some cases local steroid injections may be required.

It is helpful to give the patient an idea of the likely duration of the impediment of function caused by a sprain. For example, the time taken to recover from a sprained ankle varies from person to person, but as a guide most are noticeably better after five to seven days and fully healed at four to six weeks. Gentle walking can be resumed a few days after injury and jogging begun at two to four weeks.

SUMMARY OF MUSCULOSKELETAL DISORDERS

Achilles tendon injury

Inflammation of the Achilles tendon (tendinitis) may be a result of prolonged repeated loading and is common in athletes. It is provoked by cold weather or a change in ground surface, shoes or technique. Pain and swelling over the tendon occurs. It is treated in the acute phase by rest and cooling and later by heat. If it does not improve within a few days – **refer**.

A rupture of the Achilles tendon can be partial or complete and is relatively common in many sports. It often occurs in athletes who resume training after a period out of training. There is intense pain at the time of rupture. Walking, particularly on tiptoe, is impaired. There may be swelling or bruising over the lower leg and foot. A ruptured Achilles tendon requires medical attention – **refer.**

Ankle sprain

A sprained ankle is the most common soft tissue limb injury. It is an injury to a ligament, usually the outer lateral ligament, which attaches the fibula to the heel and foot bones on the outer side of the ankle joint. This lateral ligament is weaker than the inner (medial) ligament, which attaches the larger tibia to the heel bone on the inner side of the ankle.

Bursitis

Bursae are small sacs of fluid. Their function is to reduce friction and protect adjacent structures from pressure. They are found between bones and tendons, between two tendons and beneath the skin overlying a bone or tendon in particular parts of the body such as the hips, knees, feet, shoulders and elbows. Inflammation (bursitis) may be caused by friction (as in the Achilles tendon moving repetitively over a bursa) causing inflammation and secretion of fluid into the bursa, resulting in swelling and tenderness, leakage of calcium deposits from inflamed or degenerating tendons into an adjacent bursa, and infection, especially of superficial bursae, lying just beneath the skin in the elbows and knees. Bursitis is a painful condition and should be treated with rest and cooling, followed by heat after 48 hours. If pain or swelling is severe – **refer**.

Capsulitis

Capsulitis is inflammation of the fibrous supporting tissue surrounding the shoulder joint. If mobility is not restored with a programme of exercises (as soon as it is practical to do this), scarring and fibrosis of muscles, tendons and ligaments around the shoulder joint may occur, resulting in an inability (sometimes irreversible) to raise the arm above the head or behind the back (frozen shoulder) – **refer**.

Carpal tunnel syndrome

Where the tendons that control the movements of the hands and fingers cross the wrist, they are channelled through lubricating sheaths that cross the wrist in a narrow tunnel known as the carpal tunnel. Inflammation of the tendon sheaths at that point will reduce the space in the tunnel and compress the median nerve, which passes through it. Pain and sometimes numbness is felt in the forearm. The symptoms are often worse at night. The syndrome requires rest, NSAIDs, splinting and occasionally either steroids (by local or systemic injection) or surgery to release the tendon sheaths – **refer**.

Cervical spondylosis

Cervical spondylosis is degeneration of the cervical spine, similar to osteoarthritis. In the early stages, X-rays can be normal. Nerve entrapment can occur.

(continued overleaf)

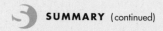 **SUMMARY** (continued)

Coccygitis

Injury to the small spur of the vertebrae at the tip of the spine (coccyx), as in a fall, causes a painful coccydinia and inflammation of the ligaments attached to the coccyx. Pain may last for several months. The best treatment is with analgesics but the long duration of the symptoms should be borne in mind. It does not normally require referral, but if there is any doubt about the diagnosis in severe cases – **refer**.

Cramp

Muscle cramp is a common condition affecting active people during strenuous exercise as well as the inactive usually at rest and those with impaired peripheral circulation (claudication). The cause is unknown, although it is thought to be due to an accumulation of lactic acid. Immediate treatment is to rest the limb, although the spasm of nocturnal cramp may be helped by weight bearing and by applying massage to stimulate the circulation. If persistent or recurrent – **refer**.

Golfer's elbow

The lower end of the humerus broadens into two bony protrusions (epicondyles). One is located on the inner (medial) side of the elbow and one on the outer (lateral) side. The epicondyles are the points of insertion of the forearm muscles that move the fingers and wrist. The muscles are joined to the epicondyles by narrow tendons. Considerable force to, and vibration in, the muscles, as in some sports or some occupations, can cause disruption of the tendons from the epicondyles. Symptoms are pain and tenderness in the inner aspect of the elbow, which may radiate along the forearm. The wrist is weak and simple clenching movements of the hand are painful. If mild, the condition responds to rest and analgesics or NSAIDs, but symptoms can take weeks or months to resolve. In more painful presentations, local steroid injections may be required. If severe – **refer**.

Lumbago

Lumbago is low back pain, most common in the third and fourth decades. It can be caused by strains of the spinal muscles and ligaments (soft tissue lumbago) or more seriously by disorders of the vertebrae, intervertebral discs and their associated joints. If the intervertebral discs are squeezed outwards and prolapse (slipped disc), there will be sudden severe backache. The patient will hold himself or herself rigid to avoid movement and will find sitting down painful and difficult. Such cases require rest.

The decision to refer depends on the course of previous episodes, but in cases where prolapse is suspected – **refer**.

Osteoarthritis

Osteoarthritis is degeneration and excessive wear of the cartilage covering the surface of bones in a joint. Its incidence is greater in the elderly. Osteoarthritis may be primary (cause unknown) or secondary (due to injury or an inappropriate load on a joint). There is joint pain, tenderness, swelling, reduced mobility and stiffness – **refer**.

→

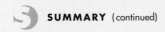 **SUMMARY** (continued)

Plantar fasciitis
The plantar fascia comprises two arch ligaments and a band of fibrous tissue overlying them, and runs over the heel bone (where it forms the heel cushion) to the toes. Stretching of the fascia can cause inflammation resulting in pain and stiffness in the sole and heel. It can be treated with rest, anti-inflammatory measures and, if necessary, arch supports. If treatment fails – **refer**.

Rheumatoid arthritis
Rheumatoid arthritis is a chronic inflammatory condition of the synovial membrane in joints, causing inflammation, pain, swelling and reduced mobility. It may also affect soft tissues such as tendons, tendon sheaths, muscles and bursae. If suspected – **refer**.

Sciatica
Sciatica is often caused by a prolapsed disc that compresses the roots of the sciatic nerve. It may be preceded by lumbago in some cases. Pain radiates from the back down one leg and there may be numbness and weakness of the leg. The back of the leg, from the buttock down the thigh as far as the calf, is the most commonly affected area, but the front of the leg can also be involved. The best treatment is rest, analgesics or NSAIDs, and heat. If the pain is severe and persists for more than a few days – **refer**.

Sprain
A sprain is an injury to a ligament or joint capsule usually caused by a forceful movement. It is characterised by pain, swelling and some loss of function.

Strain
A strain is an injury to a muscle usually caused by excessive stretching or overuse.

Tennis elbow
Tennis elbow is caused by excessive force acting on the insertion of the tendons of the forearm muscles at the outer (lateral) epicondyle (see golfer's elbow). This is common in racquet sports and also in activities involving repetitive twisting movements, such as turning a screwdriver. Symptoms are similar to those of golfer's elbow, but pain is felt in the outer part of the forearm and may spread to the upper arm. The pain is worse when the hand is clenched or is bent backwards at the wrist.

   The course of the condition is similar to that of golfer's elbow and the indications for referral are the same.

Tenosynovitis
Tenosynovitis is a painful inflammation of the muscles, tendons and tendon sheaths. It commonly occurs in the forearm. It often results from overusage (as in the popularly named pudding stirrer's thumb) and produces pain and tenderness in the flexor muscles of the forearm. It is easily confused with carpal tunnel syndrome (see above) but the latter is usually more recurrent and chronic. Treatment involves a sling to rest the arm or wrist. If this support is ineffective, a splint or even a plaster cast can be used – **refer**.

Wry neck
Wry neck (torticollis) is a painful condition in which there is spasm of one or more muscles in the neck. It occurs after straining muscles with repeated or unaccustomed movement, or on exposure to cold.

   There will be pain in the neck, sometimes extending to the top inner edge of the scapula, triggered by neck movement. The neck is tender and tense. Treatment should involve immobilisation of the neck, as far as is convenient, and analgesia. If there is no improvement in one week or if the pain is severe – **refer**.

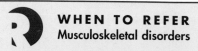

WHEN TO REFER
Musculoskeletal disorders

- There have been substantial impact forces and a fracture cannot be ruled out

- There is pain at rest

- Pain is not being relieved by OTC medicines

- Improvement in function of the affected limb is not obvious in five to seven days

- Patient is elderly or a child

- There is a bony abnormality or tenderness (by observation or touch)

- The patient cannot weight bear for four steps

- There is obvious deformity

CASE STUDIES

Case 1

The pharmacist overhears a woman asking the pharmacy assistant for two crepe bandages. The pharmacy sells a variety of dressings but in this case there is a discussion about the size suitable for a child of eight. The pharmacist offers advice, and is told the child has just tripped on a paving stone and twisted her ankle. Perhaps, the pharmacist ventures, it would be as well to have a look at it. This is not possible, the girl is resting at home and although she can weight bear it is painful, and she is limping.

The pharmacist immediately advises that a medical opinion is sought. The mother replies that the wait in the local accident and emergency department is often several hours and it will take longer than that to see her doctor, who has no X-ray facility. In any case, the girl cannot have broken anything as she was able to hobble home.

The danger, the pharmacist advises, is her youth. It does seem unlikely she has fractured anything, but the pharmacist stresses how important it is that the ankle heals properly. While admitting that the accident department will probably do no more than the mother could do herself, they will be able to assess the extent of the injury and by careful follow-up ensure no residual weakness persists. If physiotherapy, for instance, is needed they know when to initiate it.

By the time the pharmacist has finished the mother is more than convinced, and goes next door to the newsagent on her way home to buy a magazine and some chocolate as rewards for the wait ahead.

→

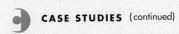

CASE STUDIES (continued)

Case 2

The pharmacist is intrigued by a man in his 40s who limps into the pharmacy sporting a substantial bandage around his ankle and a walking stick. His family watches with amusement from the pavement. The story unfolds that as a favour he offered to exercise his daughter's dog, a young but large rumbustious animal that waits impatiently outside. No doubt as a sign of affection, the dog ran into him from behind, knocking him over and then adding to the injury by jumping onto his prostrate body. The lateral malleolus is painful and very swollen, although a visit to the casualty department confirmed it was not broken. The paracetamol the hospital provided rapidly ran out, and he wonders whether anything more powerful would be suitable.

A fortnight later the man returns, requesting more of the same. The analgesics certainly provide relief, and although he is walking now without the stick, the ankle is still very painful by the end of the day. Uncomplimentary comments are made about the dog.

A further two weeks elapse before the man again appears, his tone this time rather more earnest. He needs analgesia again, but is concerned about his apparent lack of progress. The ankle, now free of bandaging, is still a little swollen beneath the malleolus. The pharmacist, quite rightly, is concerned. The original injury, even without fracture, is significant. The disability at the time confirms that. The degree of swelling suggests a partial disruption, or avulsion, of the lateral ligament, which needs to be treated with respect. The joint is potentially unstable as a result and a further injury must be avoided. The supportive bandage should therefore be replaced and a lighter but strong proprietary support is recommended. The time-scale of the injury is also discussed. Just because there is no fracture it cannot be assumed that resolution will occur in the 10 to 14 days associated with the healing of a simple strain. The injury has affected strong weight-bearing structures, which will take weeks, possibly months, to heal.

The man returns for repeated, although less frequent, analgesia and a further ankle support four months after the original injury. The first support has worn out and a new one is needed for walking long distances – with a golf trolley, not the dog.

Case 3

A woman in her mid 70s asks to speak to the pharmacist. She is in some discomfort after a fall a few days ago, which bruised her back and hip. It did not feel too painful at first but is getting worse. Living alone, mobility is all important to her.

The probabilities of any fracture seem remote, from both the story and her ability to walk now. Yet she is frail, and at risk from a further accident. Also she is of short stature and slim, and the possibility of osteoporosis occurs to the pharmacist. She has no obvious kyphosis, and the pharmacist declines to enquire into her menopausal history, but tactfully suggests that while the pharmacist is pleased to help with her pain, a word with the doctor or nurse would be advisable, 'Just for a check up.'

The woman returns some two weeks later. The bruising has resolved, but her visit to the surgery was most interesting. They have a new bone-scanning machine, and having performed a scan on her feel she is on the borderline of osteoporosis. She has had dietary advice and some calcium and vitamin tablets while fuller investigations are performed.

'Do you know', she says, 'they asked me if I wanted to go on HRT. At my age!'

12

Skin disorders: face and scalp

Skin disorders on the face are usually relatively easy to diagnose and classify simply by observation of the lesion and by collecting information from the history. Relatively few scalp disorders will be seen by pharmacists and again it will not be difficult to differentiate them into those suitable for self-medication and those that require medical attention.

Assessing symptoms

Site

The lesions found on the face and scalp that are discussed in this chapter are shown in Table 12.1.

Types of lesion and appearance of the rash

The appearance of the lesions of acne vulgaris is well known, with the characteristic red papular lesions, pustules and blackheads. These are located particularly on the skin of the forehead, nose, chin and beard area, but can affect any part of the face. The skin is generally greasy in appearance. Acne usually appears during adolescence (see Figure 12.16) and gradually disappears in young adulthood, but it may persist in adulthood in some cases. The condition can be caused by drugs (Table 12.2).

By contrast, an acneform rash appearing during middle age may be acne rosacea (Figure 12.1). This starts as a red rash or flushing, particularly over the cheeks and bridge of the nose. It often progresses to a papular acne-like rash. The rash may appear symmetrically and is often described as a butterfly rash because of its shape and distribution. If this condition is suspected, the patient should be referred for appropriate antibiotic treatment.

Another rash that causes a butterfly appearance over the nose and cheeks is that of systemic lupus erythematosus (Figure 12.2). This is a relatively rare condition, sometimes precipitated by drugs, in which the lesions are more scaly than in rosacea. Drugs associated with this disorder include beta-blockers, chlorpromazine, hydralazine, isoniazid, lithium, methyldopa, penicillamine, phenytoin, procainamide, sulfasalazine and thiouracils.

Table 12.1 Face and scalp lesions

Face	Seborrhoeic eczema
Acne vulgaris	Shingles
Acne rosacea	Sycosis barbae
Cellulitis and erysipelas	Urticaria
Eczema – atopic, allergic, irritant	
Furuncles (boils)	**Scalp**
Cold sores	Scalp ringworm
Impetigo	Alopecia
Lupus erythematosus	Head lice
Photosensitivity	Psoriasis
Rodent ulcer	Seborrhoea capitis and dandruff

Table 12.2 Examples of drugs causing acne

Isoniazid	Phenobarbital
Lithium	Phenytoin
Oral contraceptives	Steroids

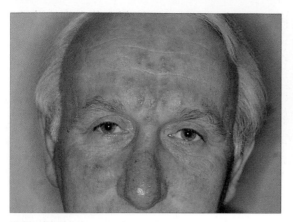

Figure 12.1 Rosacea. (Reproduced by permission from the Science Photo Library.)

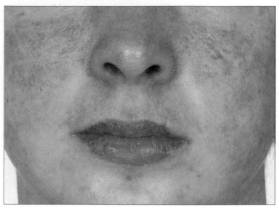

Figure 12.2 Systemic lupus erythematosus. (Reproduced with permission from the Wellcome Trust Medical Photographic Library.)

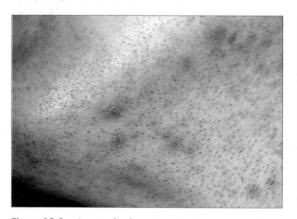

Figure 12.3 Sycosis barbae. (Reproduced with permission from the Science Photo Library.)

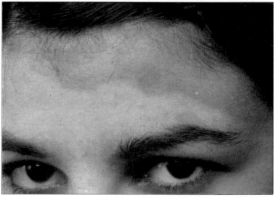

Figure 12.4 Seborrhoeic eczema. (Reproduced with permission from the Wellcome Trust Medical Photographic Library.)

Mitral valve disease, another relatively rare condition, may also be associated with a butterfly rash. In summary, any rash with a butterfly distribution over the face should be referred for a medical opinion.

The presence of red papules or pustules in the beard area is characteristic of a staphylococcal infection of the hair follicles called sycosis barbae (Figure 12.3). It may sometimes be caused by a tinea (ringworm) infection. It is most commonly seen in middle-aged men. Mild cases may resolve if shaving is stopped for a few days, but failure to resolve requires referral.

A scaly rash with mild erythema affecting the scalp and forehead, eyebrows, nose and pinna of the ear will probably be seborrhoeic eczema (Figure 12.4). It may also be associated with scaling on the edge of the eyelids (blepharitis), sometimes with loss of eyelashes. In babies during the first few months of life, it may present as cradlecap, producing yellowish crusts, chiefly on the scalp but sometimes also on the ears and eyebrows (see Figure 12.13).

A red, dry scaly rash appearing on the cheeks of babies will probably be atopic eczema (Figure 12.5). It often spreads to flexures in the neck, wrists, elbows and behind the knees. It is very irritant and the scratching that ensues can cause marked excoriation of the skin and increases the risk of infection. In older children and adults,

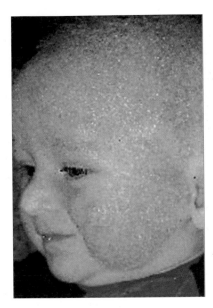

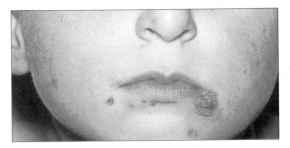

Figure 12.6   Impetigo. (Reproduced with permission from the Wellcome Trust Medical Photographic Library.)

Figure 12.5   Atopic eczema. (Reproduced with permission from the Wellcome Trust Medical Photographic Library.)

atopic eczema appears as lichenification, which is a dry, crusty thickening of the skin that often becomes cracked.

Erythema around the nose and mouth with vesicles that weep and then produce yellow or brown crusty scabs suggests impetigo (Figure 12.6). This occurs most commonly in children during the early school years. It may be difficult to differentiate from infective eczema in some cases, although the crusts of impetigo are very characteristic. In either case, a referral is necessary.

Lesions on the lips may be caused by infection with the herpes simplex virus, which causes cold sores. These are often self-diagnosed by the patient. There is usually a tingling or pricking sensation in the early stages and it is at this time that treatment with OTC medication should be started for best effect.

A tender, red swollen area of skin may herald a furuncle (boil), which is an abscess with a single pus-filled or discharging centre. Boils are commonly seen on the nose or chin, but can also occur on the nape of the neck, particularly in adolescent males. Sometimes such a red area may be the result of an insect bite and, rarely, it will be a streptococcal or staphylococcal skin infection called cellulitis (Figure 12.7).

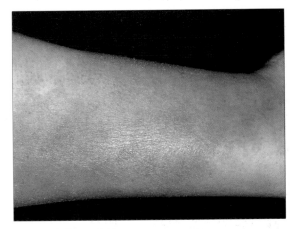

Figure 12.7   Cellulitis. (Reproduced with permission from the Medical Slide Library.)

Large urticarial weals should be observed with caution. If there is any suggestion that they are spreading quickly and becoming confluent or if they are accompanied by swelling of the eyelids or lips (angioedema), the patient should be referred swiftly to an accident and emergency department.

A small, discrete, raised nodular lesion that eventually ruptures to form a small, red or purple wart-like ulcer should be viewed with suspicion, since this is the way in which rodent ulcers (basal cell carcinoma) present (Figure 12.8). They can occur anywhere on the face but are most common on the nose, cheeks and pinna of the ear. Any suspicion requires a referral.

A raised cystic lump of epidermis may be due to a sebaceous cyst, which is most commonly

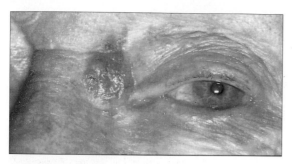

Figure 12.8   Rodent ulcer. (Reproduced with permission from the Royal Victoria Infirmary, Newcastle upon Tyne.)

found on the face, ears or neck. It appears as a pale, non-pigmented, firm swelling and is painless, but requires referral to confirm the diagnosis. The only remedy, if the lesion is upsetting to the patient, is surgery.

A yellow discoloration of the skin of the face should be suspected as jaundice. This can be confirmed by observing a similar discoloration of the sclera of the eyes. Referral is necessary for a medical opinion. Jaundice may not necessarily represent a serious disorder.

A facial rash resembling sunburn that is limited to exposed skin on the face, neck and possibly the backs of the hands suggests a photosensitive rash. This is often caused by drugs (see Table 12.3). A

striking slate blue or grey discoloration of the face is characteristically caused by amiodarone. Questioning of the patient about current medication is therefore important. Although the use of a sunblock and advice to cover the skin are helpful, the patient should be referred initially.

Vitiligo is a condition in which lack of pigmentation occurs in small, irregularly shaped areas of the skin anywhere on the face as well as on the neck and limbs (Figure 12.9). This condition is caused by a lack, or destruction, of melanocytes. It is generally harmless, although the lesions will tend to sunburn more than the surrounding skin. In rare cases, vitiligo is associated with other diseases such as pernicious anaemia, thyroid disorders and diabetes, and therefore the patient should be advised to see a doctor in the initial stages so that any complications can be excluded.

Contact eczema on the face most commonly occurs around the eyes (often caused by allergens in cosmetics) or on the pinna of the ears (caused by allergy to nickel in earrings; Figure 12.10). It may, however, be seen anywhere on the face, according to the irritant or sensitising agent used. It occurs as an erythematous rash, with inflammation. On the ears in particular, weeping vesicles are often seen which eventually produce crusting lesions.

Isolated, small punctate red macules (called naevi; Figure 12.11) appearing on the face may be due to dilatation of capillaries in the skin. They may sometimes be star shaped or spider-like. One or two such lesions on the face may be

Descriptive terms used in dermatology	
Bulla	A large blister containing serum
Erythema	Redness due to inflammation
Excoriation	Marks on the skin caused by scratching
Lichenification	A thickening of the skin, often a result of rubbing in localised areas in eczema
Macule	A well-defined mark on the skin, which is flat and not raised (e.g. freckle)
Papule	A small, raised lesion – a large papule is termed a nodule
Plaque	A well-defined, raised patch of tissue (commonly seen in psoriasis)
Pustule	A small blister containing pus
Vesicle	A small blister containing serum (i.e. non-purulent)

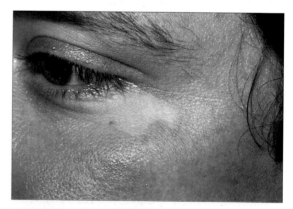

Figure 12.9   Vitiligo. (Reproduced with permission from Dr Chris Hale/Science Photo Library.)

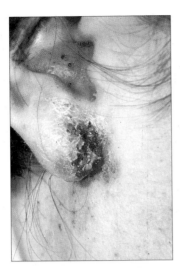

Figure 12.10   Reaction to nickel. (Reproduced with permission from the Wellcome Trust Medical Photographic Library.)

Figure 12.12   Telangiectasia. (Reproduced with permission from the Wellcome Trust Medical Photographic Library.)

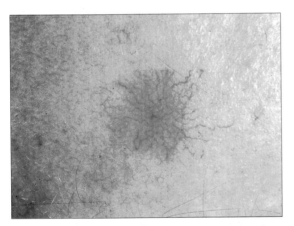

Figure 12.11   Spider naevus. (Reproduced with permission from the Royal Victoria Infirmary, Newcastle upon Tyne.)

quite normal. The lesions are so small that they are often not noticed but if they increase in number their presence may be detected by the patient. The red spot will blanch for one or two seconds when pressure is applied from a finger. They are common in pregnancy and in women taking combined oral contraceptives and there is no need to refer unless the patient is particularly anxious. Other causes include liver disease and therefore any other symptoms such as general malaise, jaundiced skin or sclera, or the suspicion of a high alcohol intake should alert the

pharmacist to advise the patient to seek a medical opinion.

A more striking dilatation of small blood vessels in the face, telangiectasia (Figure 12.12), is more common in the elderly and often occurs as a result of age-related thinning of the supporting structures of the dermis. A network of red or purple veins is visible through a relatively thin or translucent skin. In the elderly it causes no symptoms other than cosmetic unacceptability in some patients and generally requires no treatment. The condition is often associated with acne rosacea in the middle aged.

Seborrhoea capitis presents as dandruff and an itchy scalp, and is associated with seborrhoeic eczema elsewhere on the skin, blepharitis and acne. In babies, it presents as cradlecap (see Figure 12.13).

One of the most common causes of an itchy scalp, especially in children, is head lice. Infection can be suspected by visual evidence of the white egg cases (nits), which lodge onto the hairs. The nits are initially found close to the scalp, although they may be seen further away from the scalp as the affected hair grows. The diagnosis of head lice infection can, however, only be made when lice are detected by combing dampened hair with a fine tooth comb over a sheet of white paper. Outbreaks of head lice often occur in schools, nurseries, etc., and parents will often diagnose the condition themselves. Treatment and prophylaxis can be undertaken with

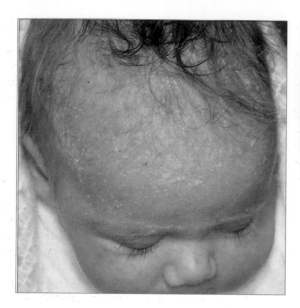

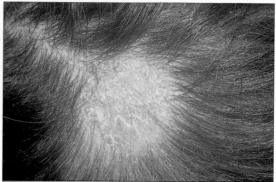

Figure 12.14   Tinea capitis.

Figure 12.13   Cradlecap. (Reproduced with permission from the Wellcome Trust Medical Photographic Library.)

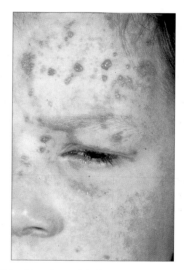

Figure 12.15   Shingles ophthalmic. (Reproduced with permission from the Wellcome Trust Medical Photographic Library.)

appropriate OTC medication. More details of head lice infection appear in Chapter 14.

A bald patch on the scalp may be caused either by alopecia areata or by scalp ringworm (tinea capitis; Figure 12.14). The latter tends to present as scaly itching lesions, the former without scales and with no irritation. Both should be referred, if suspected.

Severe scaling of the scalp may be due to psoriasis. Psoriasis rarely affects the face, but it may be found elsewhere on the body, giving a clue to the diagnosis of any scalp lesions. On the scalp it usually appears as a scaly or red rash and there may be some loss of hair.

A rash occurring unilaterally over the scalp and forehead, extending to the eye, should be suspected as shingles (Figure 12.15). The rash may be macular at first, changing to vesicles and it can be very painful. The patient should be referred immediately.

Duration and onset

Many skin conditions are chronic and the patient will report a long-standing lesion or rash. In such cases, time is not of the essence and even if referral is thought to be appropriate, it can be arranged at the patient's convenience in most cases. Examples of such conditions are acne vulgaris and rosacea, seborrhoea, most cases of eczema, vitiligo, telangiectasia, psoriasis and even a suspected rodent ulcer, although in the last case the importance of seeing a doctor should be emphasised to the patient. More acute situations will require more urgent referral, the timescale depending on the severity of the signs and symptoms. Thus, infections such as cellulitis and drug-related photosensitivity may need an opinion within a day or two, whereas angioedema or jaundice, particularly where the patient has other significant symptoms or is feeling unwell, require more urgent attention.

Angioedema should be regarded as a medical emergency.

The onset of a skin rash can often be related in time to likely causative factors, such as the use of a hair colourant or cosmetics, or concomitant drug therapy.

Reference has already been made to the age of the patient, which may give some clue as to the likelihood of particular diagnoses. Thus, acne vulgaris usually starts in adolescence and generally has disappeared by young adulthood. Impetigo and head lice are less likely to be seen in adults than young children.

Accompanying symptoms

Swelling of the lips or tongue, especially in the case of an urticarial rash, requires immediate medical attention.

Itching (pruritus) is a common accompaniment to eczema and also to scalp infections and infestations. Generalised itching over most of the body without the appearance of a rash may be a sign of systemic disease, such as liver or kidney disease, and the patient should be referred. Headache, fever, malaise and lymphadenopathy (swollen glands, seen or felt easily in the neck) suggest systemic disease or infection and require referral.

Spread

Acne vulgaris, although occurring most noticeably on the face, is often found also on the neck, upper chest and back. In acne rosacea there may eventually be involvement of the nose, resulting in rhinophyma, in which the nose becomes enlarged, rounded and red.

Photosensitivity rashes will be seen on other sites exposed to light, besides the face, such as the backs of the hands, neck and upper chest. Non-photosensitive drug rashes will often appear as a morbilliform rash, usually involving the trunk and sometimes the limbs, as well as the face.

The rashes of measles and German measles (rubella) characteristically begin on the face or the back of the neck and spread down the trunk. Psoriasis and eczema both appear on other parts

of the body. Psoriasis occurs usually as individual plaques of scaly, silvery lesions, particularly on the knees, elbows and forearms. Eczema may be localised to sites where there is contact with irritants or sensitising agents, and atopic eczema to sites where there are flexures in the skin, such as the wrists, behind the knees and the elbows.

Recurrence

Some skin lesions will recur after a relatively symptom-free interval. This may represent a chronic condition that spontaneously resolves and relapses (e.g. seborrhoeic eczema or atopic eczema), repeated exposure to the chemical irritant or allergen (as may occur in contact irritant or allergic eczema) or re-infection and re-infestation from close human contact (e.g. impetigo or head lice).

Repeated bacterial infections, such as boils or cellulitis, can occur in patients with diabetes. Patients with this condition should be questioned about their blood glucose control while those who have never been diagnosed as having diabetes should be questioned about the presence of nocturia, thirst and weight loss.

Management

Eczema

Emollient creams and ointments are useful to hydrate the skin and form an occlusive barrier to prevent further evaporation of moisture. This action is particularly appropriate in dry lesions, such as atopic eczema on the face. Non-proprietary preparations such as aqueous cream and oily cream are suitable and there is also an array of proprietary emollient products.

If irritants or sensitising agents are thought to be the cause of an eczematous reaction, it is obvious that these should be removed or the skin protected from them before any treatment is going to be successful. In the case of sensitivity to nickel earrings, proprietary lacquers are available to coat the earrings and prevent contact with the skin. Topical hydrocortisone may be applied on the ears and neck but it is not licensed for OTC use on the face.

Wet and weeping eczematous lesions can be treated with potassium permanganate soaks or compresses. These may be particularly useful when lesions are crusting and weeping. A few crystals of potassium permanganate should be dissolved in a cupful of water and the solution applied for about 15 minutes two or three times daily. The mechanism of action is not clear, but this is a traditional method used by dermatologists for treating weeping eczema.

Mild cases of seborrhoeic eczema can be treated with mild keratolytics, for example 0.5 or 1 per cent salicylic acid in a vehicle such as aqueous cream. Chronic cases or those causing skin irritation are usually best referred for a medical opinion regarding topical steroid or antifungal treatment.

Acne products

The most common constituent of proprietary creams and gels for acne treatment is benzoyl peroxide. It is bactericidal to *Propionibacterium acnes* and is thought to act in part by reducing the breakdown of sebum into irritant fatty acids, which cause inflammation in the sebaceous ducts. Benzoyl peroxide is also keratolytic and is thereby thought to unplug the ducts and drain the sebum from the sebaceous glands. It often causes dryness, erythema, peeling and stinging after the first few applications. Patients should be forewarned of this and advised to use products cautiously at first, perhaps just once a day. If usage proves to be too unpleasant, the patient should be told to stop application for a few days and then start again, perhaps on alternate days at first. Application should be to all the affected area and not just to the comedones. Benzoyl peroxide is also well known for its bleaching action on clothes and hair, and this should be pointed out to patients before use. In common with most acne remedies, there may be no apparent benefit for several weeks or months after starting treatment and it is wise to ensure that patients are aware of this. Products containing a low concentration (5 per cent) should be used at first and if no improvement is seen after four weeks, a higher concentration can be substituted.

Salicylic acid is an old established keratolytic agent which is present in various proprietary products as well as in official preparations such as salicylic acid ointment. It is thought by some to have dubious efficacy in acne and its use is falling out of favour.

Other traditional keratolytics include sulphur and potassium hydroxyquinoline and these are found in combination with benzoyl peroxide in some products.

Frequent washing and degreasing improves acne, and various cleansing lotions and skin washes are marketed for this purpose. Patients should be advised to take advantage of sunshine as this removes excess oil from the skin and appears to be beneficial.

Cold sores

Cold sores can be treated with an antiviral cream containing five per cent aciclovir. It should be applied to the lesion as early as possible, at the time that a tingling sensation is felt.

Scalp treatments

Seborrhoea capitis may be treated with an anti-dandruff shampoo, such as a product containing selenium or zinc pyrithione. Ketoconazole shampoo, which attacks the *Pityrosporum ovale* yeast, a causative factor in seborrhoea, is effective, especially in difficult cases. Tar-based shampoos may also be useful. Severe or chronic cases may need to be referred.

In babies, cradlecap can be managed by rubbing in olive oil or emulsifying ointment to loosen the scales and then shampooing out with a standard baby shampoo. Mild keratolytics, such as 0.5 per cent salicylic acid in emulsifying ointment, may also be used but care must be taken that such treatment is not undertaken on a regular basis to reduce the risk of any absorption.

Mild cases of psoriasis on the scalp can be treated with shampoos containing coal tar, but more severe cases are best referred.

The prevention and treatment of head lice is a common problem that pharmacists are asked to deal with. Firstly, there are various health education messages which are important to convey, such as eliminating the stigma that head lice are associated with a lack of hygiene or care and the view that short hair is less likely to be infested than long hair. Indeed the term 'infestation' should be replaced with 'infection' when referring to head lice, to remove the pejorative overtones that exist among the lay public. The prophylactic use of a pesticide shampoo or lotion should be discouraged as it will be largely ineffective and may give rise to resistance. Treatment of head lice can be with an anti-cholinesterase such as malathion or a pyrethroid such as phenothrin or permethrin. Treatment should be with a lotion rather than a shampoo.

Resistance to insecticidal preparations has occurred and the former practice of rotating the use of insecticides across a district has now lost favour. The current maxim 'no louse, no treatment' may help to reduce the indiscriminate use of insecticides and thereby lessen the prevalence of apparent resistance. Criteria for diagnosis of infection are described in detail in Chapter 14 and pharmacists should become more confident in confirming cases and starting treatment.

It is also important for pharmacists to educate parents about the pathogenesis of the condition, pointing out particularly that the symptom of an itchy scalp is an allergic reaction to lice. The itchiness usually manifests itself several weeks after the scalp has become infected and, in similar fashion, may not disappear until several days or weeks after all lice have been removed. Before a course of treatment with two applications of insecticide is deemed to have failed, on the whim of an anxious parent who believes that a child who persists in scratching its scalp must still be infected, evidence for the presence of lice must therefore be produced. Until detection combing produces such evidence, consideration cannot be given to further chemical treatment using other insecticides.

Full details of techniques for detection and treatment are given in Chapter 14.

 SUMMARY OF CONDITIONS PRODUCING FACE AND SCALP LESIONS

Acne vulgaris

Acne is caused by inflammation and blockage of the sebaceous glands and hair follicles. It is associated with the bacterium *Propionibacterium acnes*, which is thought to split the triglycerides in sebum into fatty acids, which are irritant to the pilosebaceous unit. The condition is recognised by the familiar comedones (blackheads), which often become pustular. There is no pruritus but the rash causes embarrassment and self-consciousness in young people. It occurs predominantly on the face but also appears on the nape of the neck, shoulders and the upper trunk. In severe cases, scarring may result. Acne is most common in adolescents (Figure 12.16), classically appearing around the time of puberty, although it can persist into adulthood.

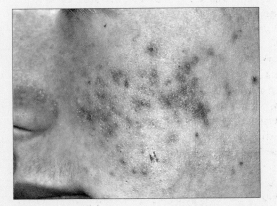

Figure 12.16   Adolescent acne vulgaris. (Reproduced with permission from Dr P. Marazzi/Science Photo Library.)

(continued overleaf)

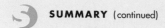 **SUMMARY** (continued)

Acne rosacea

Acne rosacea is a skin condition of uncertain origin. It appears with a characteristic pattern of flushing over the bridge of the nose and the cheeks (see Figure 12.1), often referred to as a butterfly rash, and may progress to acne-like papules – **refer**.

Allergic eczema

Contact between an allergen and the skin may produce an eczematous reaction at the site of contact and sometimes at a site distant from it. The most common examples on the head are nickel allergy (from earrings) and sensitisation to perfumes and cosmetics.

Atopic eczema

Atopy is an inherited predisposition to develop asthma, hay fever and eczema. Atopic eczema is a constitutional eczema usually occurring in patients with a family history of atopy. It commonly begins after the first few months of life and although it often resolves spontaneously it can persist into adulthood. The lesions are erythematous, papular and either dry or weeping. They are commonly seen on the face, for example on the cheeks (see Figure 12.5), and also on the wrists, arms and knee flexures. They are accompanied by intense pruritus, leading to frenzied scratching in some children.

Cellulitis

Cellulitis is a bacterial infection of the skin caused by either streptococci or staphylococci. The infection may arise at the site of trauma but it can also affect previously healthy skin. A similar condition caused by streptococci is called erysipelas. The rash is red and often hot and oedematous (see Figure 12.7). There is often headache, fever and malaise – **refer**.

Furuncles

A furuncle (boil) is a superficial abscess, usually caused by *Staphylococcus aureus*, which has a single discharging centre. Males and adolescents are most commonly affected. Furuncles are mostly sited on the face, nape of the neck, ears and nose. Patients with recurrent boils should be checked for diabetes.

Impetigo

Impetigo is a contagious bacterial infection of the epidermis caused by either staphylococci or streptococci. It mostly affects children of school age and causes a weeping, vesicular rash, which eventually dries to form yellowish brown crusted lesions (see Figure 12.6). Itching results in scratching, which leads to a spread of the infection on the skin – **refer**.

Irritant contact eczema

Irritant chemicals can cause trauma to the skin, resulting in an inflamed area at the point of contact. The most common irritants are soaps, detergents, shampoos, bleaches and various substances used in the workplace. The rash usually resolves when the irritant is removed.

Photosensitive dermatitis

Photosensitivity causes a rash with a characteristic appearance on the face, neck, back of the hands and upper chest. It may be aggravated by various drugs (Table 12.3).

→

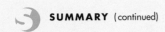

SUMMARY (continued)

Table 12.3 Examples of photosensitising drugs	
Amiodarone	Sulfonamides
Chloropromazine	Tetracyclines
Nalidixic acid	Thiazides
NSAIDs	Tricyclic antidepressants
Quinolones	

Psoriasis

Psoriatic lesions rarely occur on the face, but may be seen on the scalp and at other sites. Psoriatic plaques, recognised as red lesions covered with silvery scales, may be found on the elbows, knees and the lower back. On the scalp the lesions appear as a thick mat of dandruff, with loss of hair. It is a chronic recurrent disorder – **refer**.

Scalp ringworm

Scalp ringworm (tinea capitis) appears as a round, scaly, bald patch in and around which may be seen broken stumps of hair follicles (see Figure 12.14). Treatment is often systemic – **refer**.

Seborrhoeic eczema

Seborrhoea is a marked increase in the activity of the sebaceous glands. The yeast *Pityrosporum* has been implicated as a causative agent. It appears as dry or greasy scales affecting the skin behind the ears, the external ear canal, the fold between the nose and extremities of the mouth, the hair margin and eyebrows (see Figure 12.4). It may cause slight pruritus. It often spreads to the scalp (seborrhoea capitis), where it is characterised by scaly dandruff and erythema of varying severity. Seborrhoea is often associated with acne, chronic blepharitis (see Chapter 5) and otitis externa (see Chapter 10).

Shingles

Shingles is caused by reactivation of the herpes zoster (chickenpox) virus which has lain dormant in a sensory root ganglion. Skin lesions follow the course of sensory nerves. The infection is most contagious during the period before the rash appears. The rash is macular at first, then vesicular and eventually it forms crusts. It is often very painful. It can occur on the scalp, extending unilaterally over the forehead and eye (see Figure 12.15). There may be fever, malaise and anorexia before the rash appears. There is often a painful neuralgia that persists for many weeks after the rash has disappeared – **refer**.

Spider naevi

Spider naevi are small capillary dilatations that may be punctate, stellate or spider shaped (see Figure 12.11). They characteristically blanch when pressure is applied. They are most common on the face but can occur on the trunk. Isolated spider naevi are not unusual in healthy people and increased numbers can appear in pregnancy or in women taking oral contraceptives. They may appear in significant numbers in liver disease and if this is suspected – **refer**. Generally there is no treatment.

(continued overleaf)

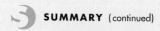 **SUMMARY** (continued)

Sycosis barbae and tinea barbae

These two conditions are due to staphylococcal and tinea infection, respectively. They are characterised by a crusted, raised, pustular folliculitis in the beard area (see Figure 12.3), which is exacerbated by shaving – **refer**.

Telangiectasia

Telangiectasia is a dilatation of superficial blood vessels in the skin (see Figure 12.12). It may be inherited in some cases and can also be caused by potent topical steroids, ageing, prolonged exposure to the sun and certain systemic diseases such as systemic lupus erythematosus. Referral is not necessary unless a serious condition is suspected.

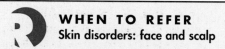 **WHEN TO REFER**
Skin disorders: face and scalp

- Small discrete ulcer or lesion with raised edge (rodent ulcer)
- Any severe condition that does not respond to OTC management, such as eczema, seborrhoeic eczema, dandruff and acne
- Papular rash, with or without vesicles and crusting, in the beard area of men
- Vesicles or crusting rash indicating infection
- Rash around the mouth or nose of children that changes to weeping vesicles, eventually forming yellow crusts
- Butterfly distribution of erythema over the nose and cheeks
- Any newly appeared lump, even without symptoms such as itch or pain
- Abnormal facial coloration, such as yellow, blue or greyish complexion, or a sun-tanned appearance, extending to the whole body, when there is no history of sun exposure (as may occur in the hyper-pigmentation that accompanies suppression of the adrenal glands)
- Small, discrete, red macular lesions that blanch when pressure is applied with a finger
- Small thread-like veins in the skin, especially on the cheeks – not a reason for referral unless the patient is anxious or receiving steroid medication either orally or topically
- Abnormal hair loss, not related to male-pattern hair loss
- Unilateral rash on the face, scalp or the skin around the eye, especially if it is painful
- Acne, photosensitive rash or yellow, jaundiced skin coloration that has recently appeared or has been exacerbated in a patient taking any medication that could be responsible
- Rash on the face that spreads down to the trunk

→

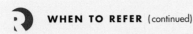

WHEN TO REFER (continued)

Accompanying symptoms
- Any facial lesion accompanied by any of the following: malaise, fever, headache or swollen lymph glands in the neck
- Swelling of the eyelids or lips, or difficulty with breathing – emergency referral to hospital
- Refer all diabetic patients with signs or symptoms of skin infection, especially if recurrent, such as boils or cellulitis

---

CASE STUDIES

Case 1

The man in the pharmacy is well known to the pharmacist. He is in his early 60s and has worked as a builder all his life. He has well-controlled diabetes, in part at least due to moderate obesity, and comes in regularly with prescriptions for his oral hypoglycaemics. A rugged, outdoor man, he wears his hair long, often with a cap on top, but sometimes revealing a nodular lesion on the pinna of his right ear. On one occasion this is covered with an awkward plaster. The pharmacist, never having mentioned it before, enquires and is told it is nothing more than a wart that has been there for years and is of no consequence.

At the next visit the lesion is revealed, and the pharmacist remarks on it. On close inspection it is a rounded pearly lesion that is dimpled in its centre. A basal cell carcinoma is suspected and medical referral is urged. The pharmacist remains doubtful whether this advice will be followed, and so is pleased to learn that it was, although subsequently the patient remonstrates with the pharmacist as the hospital talk of radiotherapy, skin grafts and much more, and clearly the removal of his wart will cost him dearly.

However, with his next three-monthly prescription, the man has a different story. The offending lesion has gone, his ear looks normal and above all he is full of thanks. It was after all a cancer, which but for the intervention of the pharmacist would almost certainly by now have engulfed him. A half-hearted explanation that this condition never metastasises and must be the safest malignancy known falls, as it were, on deaf ears but secures a promise to take a look at the leaking flat roof over the dispensary at the back of the pharmacy within the week.

Case 2

A slightly overweight woman in her mid 50s presents the pharmacist with a new prescription for a thiazide diuretic. She has been seeing the practice nurse for a 'well person check', and repeated blood pressure measurements have been marginally elevated.

The pharmacist begins the usual explanations in this circumstance, but quickly realises the woman is paying no attention, her mind being elsewhere. The pharmacist stops in mid sentence and the woman apologises. On her last visit to the nurse she mentioned a rash over her nose and cheeks, which although disguised with make-up is bothering her somewhat. She was fairly abruptly told it was most likely due to

(continued overleaf)

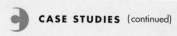

excessive alcohol intake. She enjoys a glass of wine with her husband over their evening meal, and occasionally a sherry with her mother at weekends. Even so, her total alcohol intake is well below the recommended maximum and, the pharmacist suggests, does not seem to be the likely culprit.

Encouraged by this news, and using a tissue to remove the camouflage, a red, thickened area of skin is revealed in a butterfly distribution over the bridge of her nose. The pharmacist reassures her that while a definitive diagnosis cannot be given in the pharmacy, diagnosis and treatment can be obtained from her doctor.

The pharmacist is rewarded a week later when the woman presents a prescription for low-dose antibiotics.

'Rosacea', she proclaims with some satisfaction.

The pharmacist attempts to counter this, as her prescription charge is taken, by explaining she will probably need long-term treatment.

'Yes,' she agrees, 'but just think what I'll save on cosmetics.'

Case 3

A man in his early 60s comes in and asks for something for migraine. He has never had it before, although for two days he has had a constant but increasing pain over the left temple and side of his face, with odd sensations of tingling and hot and cold. With no nausea or visual disturbance the pharmacist questions this diagnosis. Sinus problems, temporal arteritis and other possibilities are probed but seem unlikely. Finally an analgesic is purchased, although the pharmacist would prefer referral to the doctor. This is impossible, the man says, for today is Friday and he is going on holiday the following week.

The next day the man's wife calls in for sun cream. Still uneasy about the previous day, the pharmacist asks after her husband. She in turn reports the pain is worse, and there is now an erythematous rash appearing. The pharmacist is adamant. Weekend or not, he must contact the doctor.

The wife appears again when the pharmacy opens on Sunday with a prescription for antiviral therapy. Herpes zoster has been confirmed, but has been discovered in time to be treated. He also has an appointment at hospital in a couple of days. For two weeks they are frequent visitors to the pharmacy for both topical and systemic treatments associated with the shingles. Their holiday has had to be postponed, but even this seems a minor problem. The rash developed and could have threatened to involve the left eye, with the prospect of many months of pain and possible blindness with it. As it was, this did not happen, due at least in part to early intervention by the pharmacist and the persistent advice to seek a medical opinion.

13

Skin disorders: trunk and limbs

Assessing symptoms

Location and spread

Hands and arms

The hands are particularly susceptible to traumatic or contact irritant eczema. Common irritants include detergents, mineral oils and various degreasing agents. The backs of the hands and fingers are often affected first, as the skin here is less protected than on the palms, but if the irritant is being gripped or held (e.g. tools) the eczema appears on the palm. In cases of contact eczema caused by immersion of the hands in an irritant, such as washing-up liquid, both hands will be affected. The skin will usually appear red and will be sore.

An eczematous reaction caused by contact with sensitising agents, such as dyes, cement or rubber gloves, may involve the palms, depending on the specific site of contact with the skin. Psoriasis may occur as red lesions on the palms and is difficult to distinguish from chronic eczema at this site.

Lesions on the palms of the hands appearing as vesicles (small blisters) are characteristic of pompholyx (Figure 13.1), an endogenous condition (i.e. not caused by specific irritant agents or chemicals). Pompholyx often affects the feet too. The condition is very itchy and can be chronic or recurrent. If the pruritus is severe, referral is advisable for topical steroids to be considered.

Itching in the finger webs with discrete small red lesions is a classical symptom of scabies (Figure 13.2). The lesions may spread to the palms, wrists, armpits, genitalia, buttocks and abdomen. The itching is worse at night. Burrows

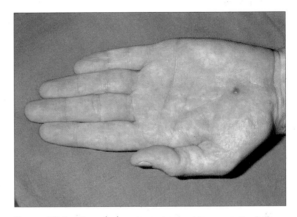

Figure 13.1 Pompholyx. (Reproduced with permission from Dr P. Marazzi/Science Photo Library.)

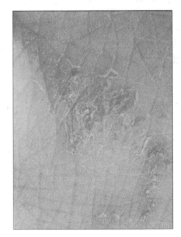

Figure 13.2 Scabies skin infection. (Reproduced with permission from the Wellcome Trust Medical Photographic Library.)

(tracks made by the mite burrowing through the skin) may be identified as small (up to 1 cm) grey curved lines in the skin, but it is not always possible to see them. Family members and any sexual contacts will sometimes also be affected.

Wrists and elbows

Besides being a site for scabies, the wrists are also common site for allergies to watch straps or nickel in jewellery.

The outside of the elbows is a common site for the characteristic appearance of psoriasis as red plaques with silvery scales (Figure 13.3).

Fingernails

Psoriasis can affect the fingernails, producing characteristic pitting or denting on the surface of the nail (Figure 13.4). This may be ignored for some time by the sufferer, who often does not associate the nail lesion with the psoriasis that is affecting the skin elsewhere. It is relatively difficult to treat and requires referral.

Fungal nail infection (onychomycosis) may present itself as painful inflammation in the skin around the base of the nails as well as involvement of the nail itself. It affects one or two nails initially but can spread to involve others. It may progress so that the nail appears thickened or yellow, although this appearance is more common in toenails. Topical antifungal agents may be effective and should be tried as a first-line treatment in mild cases in normally immuno-competent patients. However, in susceptible groups such as diabetic and immunocompromised patients, and in more severe cases, early referral is recommended to avoid complications so that oral antifungal agents can be prescribed if appropriate.

A paronychia (whitlow) is similar to onychomycosis, but is usually caused by candidal infection and affects chiefly the skin around the base of the nail. Paronychia tend to be more acute and have pus in them, which may require draining.

The appearance of the fingernail may be changed with no known, or at least no significant, cause. For example, white spots on fingernails are traditionally associated by the lay person with dietary deficiencies such as calcium, etc. This is not the case and the cause is more likely to be normal wear and tear. Patients should be given reassurance that they will grow out or lessen in time. Similarly, vertical or horizontal ridging of the nails is of little consequence, particularly in older patients, and will often disappear over several months, provided the nail is not thickened and horny (onychogryposis).

Trauma to the nail bed can produce a black nail, which is a haematoma or bruise under the nail. It will clear in time although the damaged nail may eventually separate as the new nail grows. Occasionally it may be necessary for the doctor to bore a hole in the nail to drain the blood and fluid beneath if the pressure caused by the inflammatory process is causing pain that does not disappear over a few days.

Splitting along the vertical axis of the nails may be caused by exposure of the nails to excess

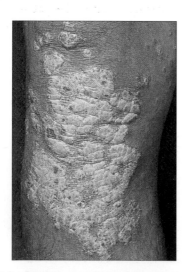

Figure 13.3   Psoriasis. (Reproduced with permission from Glaxo Wellcome.)

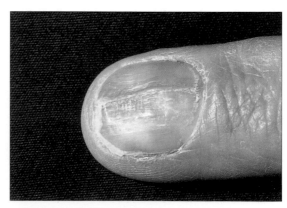

Figure 13.4   Psoriasis of the nail. (Reproduced with permission from Dr P. Marazzi/Science Photo Library.)

water or detergents, as may the condition known as 'hang nail' or ragged cuticles.

Splinter haemorrhages are rare and appear as tiny vertical dark lines in the nail. If there has been no trauma to the nail, referral is necessary since they can sometimes be a sign of systemic disease.

Feet

The foot is a site for allergic contact eczema caused by leather shoes or the dye in stockings and socks. The soles may be affected by psoriasis, which can also affect the nails. Psoriasis may be recognised by the concurrent appearance of lesions elsewhere.

Perhaps the most common skin condition affecting the feet that will present to the pharmacist is tinea pedis (athlete's foot; Figure 13.5). This usually starts between the toes (classically between the fourth and fifth digit) and can spread to the sole and upper part of the foot. It often appears red and itchy at first and later turns white with maceration and soreness between the toes. Involvement of the interdigital space helps to distinguish athlete's foot from eczematous or psoriatic conditions.

Fungal infections of the toenail may be a consequence of the spread of infection from the surrounding skin or may represent isolated lesions, as can occur in the fingernail (see above).

Other conditions affecting the feet are described in Chapter 15.

Legs

Itchy papules or larger lumps on the lower leg are often the result of insect bites, including flea bites from pets. Fleas may also attack the trunk and neck. The diagnosis can generally be confirmed by an appropriate history from the patient. If scabies can be identified elsewhere on the skin, it may manifest itself here too. Inquiry as to whether other family members are similarly affected may provide a helpful clue, although individuals react differently to insect bites.

The plaques of psoriasis (red with silvery scales) are classically seen on the knee and are quite distinctive and relatively easy to recognise. An itching rash behind the knee is likely to be atopic eczema (Figure 13.6), particularly in children.

A rash around the ankles, particularly in elderly patients, may be varicose or stasis eczema, caused by poor circulation in the lower limbs. It is often sore, dry and lichenified and may lead to oedema and eventually to leg ulcers.

Lichen planus is an eruption of small, itchy, papules which are often a purplish colour initially, later turning brown (Figure 13.7). Sometimes a white lace-like pattern may be seen on the papules. The condition often affects the mouth at the same time, producing characteristic white lacy streaks on the buccal mucosa. As well as the legs, this condition can also occur on the wrists, back and abdomen. It is usually symmetrical, occurring on both legs at similar sites. It is seen in young and middle-aged adults, but is rarer in the elderly and in children.

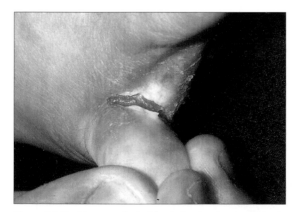

Figure 13.5 Tinea pedis (athlete's foot). (Reproduced with permission from Dr P. Marazzi/Science Photo Library.)

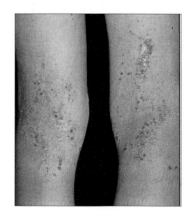

Figure 13.6 Atopic eczema. (Reproduced with permission from Glaxo Wellcome.)

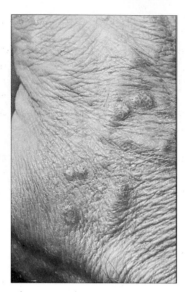

Figure 13.7   Lichen planus. (Reproduced with permission from Glaxo Wellcome.)

Skin conditions affecting the groin and genital area are generally very irritating. Scabies may appear as red papules. Pubic lice have a characteristic appearance, which leads to them being referred to as 'crabs' by the lay person. They lay eggs, in a similar way to head lice, which may be detected on pubic hair. Both scabies and pubic lice may be spread to others by close physical and sexual contact. Scabies is commonly transferred by holding hands and lice can be transferred from unwashed clothing, towels and bedlinen.

The groin is a site where intertrigo may occur. This is an eruption caused by friction between opposing folds of skin. The moist warm conditions at such sites are conducive to infection by tinea and candida. Tinea infection of the groin (tinea cruris) is relatively common, especially in men. It appears as a red, itchy rash on the inner thighs, adjacent to but rarely involving the scrotum. The rash is typical of tinea infections, with a well-defined edge that is generally redder than the centre of the lesion and spreading outwards.

The rash of candidiasis in the groin can be differentiated from tinea by its less well-defined edges; also, there are often satellite lesions (sometimes vesicular) beyond the rim of the rash.

The groin is also the site for pubic lice infection. This will usually be self-diagnosed by the patient but may be described as intense, continuous itching. Pubic lice may spread in hairy males and may even affect the eyelashes. In children without body hair, it is the scalp margins and eyelashes that are principally affected.

Trunk

Rashes that cover large areas of the body are probably best referred for a medical opinion. Sometimes the cause may be obvious, as when associated with drug treatment or when the patient is sensitive to certain foodstuffs. If urticaria appears shortly after exposure to drug or food allergens, care should be taken that swelling of the eyelids or of the tongue or airways (angioedema) does not occur. If there is any suspicion of this, the patient should be directed to a hospital casualty department as a matter of urgency. Other reactions generally require less urgent referral, but a medical opinion is desirable, if only to make the general practitioner aware of a possible adverse drug reaction so that treatment can be reviewed.

Herpes zoster infection (shingles) manifests itself as a unilateral rash, following the course of a nerve tract, which is commonly described as a belt of erythema followed by small blisters (Figure 13.8). The rash may run from the back across the chest, along the course of an intercostal nerve (between two ribs) or around the abdomen, always stopping at the midline. The condition can be very painful, both before the rash appears and after it has gone.

The plaques of psoriasis can be found in the sacral area of the back.

Tinea corporis occurs as isolated lesions or clusters of round or oval red patches on the trunk or limbs (Figure 13.9). The well-defined edges are helpful if the diagnosis is in doubt.

Vagrants and people with low standards of personal and domestic hygiene who present with severe itching may have body lice. These mites live in clothes and bedding, and bite the trunk, buttocks and shoulders. Questioning about the site of the initial skin irritation can sometimes help to distinguish this condition from scabies.

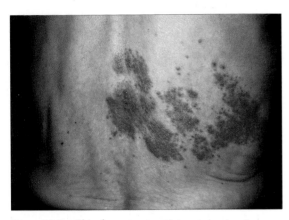

Figure 13.8 Shingles. (Reproduced with permission from the Medical Slide Library.)

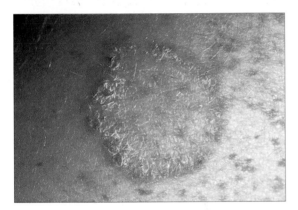

Figure 13.9 Tinea corporis (ringworm rash) on an arm. (Reproduced with permission from Dr P. Marazzi/Science Photo Library.)

with tiny discrete nodules under each sweat gland.

Another type of sweat rash may be caused by candidal infection, especially in intertriginous areas where folds of skin overlap to produce a moist, warm environment. Usual sites are under the breasts, the axillae and also the back. The groin has already been mentioned as another area that may be infected.

Although classically affecting the face, seborrhoeic eczema and acne can also affect the chest. The diagnosis can be confirmed by the presence of lesions on the face.

Duration

Skin conditions vary in timescale from a few hours to chronic disease lasting a lifetime. If a new skin condition does not show improvement within one or two weeks, then as a general rule it is wise to refer the patient. Sometimes a topical steroid will clear a mild eczema, which if otherwise left might progress to a more severe or chronic condition.

The early recognition and referral of patients with shingles will optimise the effects of therapy, which should be instigated early to reduce the unpleasant sequelae that can occur.

Accompanying symptoms

The location and appearance of a rash are the principal pointers to diagnosis. Some other factors can, however, be helpful, although their presence or absence should not be used as absolute criteria to exclude any conditions. Most rashes are accompanied by pruritus and this is particularly true for most types of eczema. Sometimes psoriasis does not itch. This may be useful when differentiating between a chronic eczema and psoriasis of the palms, or between an intertriginous psoriasis (such as in the groin) and a tinea or candidal infection at the same site.

It should be remembered that pruritus may, rarely, be a sign of systemic disease, often in the absence of a rash. Patients complaining of pruritus without an obvious skin lesion should therefore be referred. In many cases, scratching and

However, the precise diagnosis is of little consequence since the treatment is similar for both conditions.

Rashes on sun- or light-exposed areas of the limbs and trunk (e.g. upper chest and neck), in conjunction with a similar problem on the face, will suggest a possible light sensitivity reaction. This may be precipitated by drugs (see Chapter 12), or may be due to polymorphic light eruption (heat rash). The latter appears as erythema, with small macules, papules or vesicles, is very itchy and often appears during sudden exposure to hot climates, e.g. on foreign holidays.

Prickly heat or sweat rash occurs at sites where sweat ducts are occluded, particularly under clothing. The blocked follicles produce a reddened and often highly irritant skin surface, excoriation in response to pruritus may cause marks on the skin that can be mistaken for genuine lesions.

Malaise, fever or other systemic symptoms may accompany infections such as shingles and some other serious skin disorders, and such cases should be referred.

Any peeling of the skin, apart from that commonly associated with sunburn, requires referral as this may indicate an unusual or serious disorder. This should not be confused with the shedding of scales that may occur in some eczemas and psoriasis.

Onset and aggravating factors

A pertinent history can often unravel a potential causative agent for skin conditions. Examples include a patient lying on a sunbed after being prescribed a photosensitising drug, ingestion of seafood prior to the appearance of an urticarial rash, a picnic in a meadow followed by itchy red lumps on the lower legs (insect bites) or a comment that other family members have similar papular lesions and itching is worse at night (scabies).

Exposure to chemical irritants in the workplace or to contact allergens will often give a valuable clue in the diagnosis of contact eczemas. Constant wetting of the hands, as occurs in housewives, hairdressers, etc., increases susceptibility to contact eczema as well as to candidal infection and paronychia. As an adjunct to any treatment that may be given, patients should be advised to keep their hands dry by wearing rubber gloves.

Some conditions are thought to have a genetic association. Atopic eczema is a classic example of this and there may be a family history of eczema, hay fever or asthma. In patients with psoriasis, a history of the disease in another close family member is not unusual.

Recurrence

Many common skin conditions are chronic, for example eczema and psoriasis, and the disease will resolve and reappear at intervals. Patients should be warned of this.

It is important that the skin is treated with emollients in conditions where drying and fissuring may occur between the acute exacerbations. Most emollients are underused, and the frequent correct application may often reduce exacerbations and the need for other therapy.

Management

Antipruritics

Itching is a symptom that will be reduced as the skin lesion causing it is resolved. In this respect, topical steroids are powerful agents. Hydrocortisone 1 per cent will effectively reduce the inflammation and associated itching of mild eczemas and insect bites. Flea bites may be treated with topical hydrocortisone, but attention should also be drawn to the treatment of household furnishings (see Parasiticidal agents).

Topical antihistamines have fallen out of favour with dermatologists because of their tendency to cause sensitisation. However, although they should not be used in eczemas and psoriasis, they can be recommended for short-term treatment for insect bites, sunburn and urticarial eruptions, and cause problems in only a very small number of patients. Calamine lotion is a cheap, traditional antipruritic preparation and has long been used, especially for the relief of sunburn.

Sedating oral antihistamines are also useful for pruritus. They can be taken at night to relieve night-time pruritus as well as having a carry-over effect into the next day.

Emollients and topical hydrocortisone

Emollients, such as aqueous cream, emulsifying ointment and a large number of proprietary products, are extremely important agents in the treatment of chronic eczema and psoriasis. They maintain hydration of the stratum corneum by reducing evaporation and this is effective in preventing drying and cracking of the skin, which can be very painful. They should be applied after washing or bathing.

The choice between the different products available is largely one of cosmetic acceptability by the patient. Ointments such as emulsifying ointment tend to be most effective, but creams such as aqueous and proprietary creams are less greasy and more acceptable to patients. However, where dry skin is a particular problem in a non-visible part of the body, such as the feet, priority should be given to efficacy rather than cosmetic tolerance.

Eczematous patients should be discouraged from using perfumed soap and bath additives, as these may cause sensitisation as well as having a degreasing effect on the skin, causing it to dry out after bathing. Instead, a proprietary bath emollient or emulsifying ointment can be used. The latter can be used in the bath by mixing about 100 g in a bowl of hot water before adding to the bath water, or alternatively mixing this amount thoroughly, a little at a time, in the water under the tap. Most bath emollients contain light liquid paraffin as the active constituent and although their effectiveness is matched by emulsifying ointment, they tend to be more cosmetically acceptable, despite their higher cost.

OTC topical hydrocortisone 1 per cent is licensed for short-term use in the treatment of mild to moderate eczema in flare-ups in known sufferers as well as for contact eczema and insect bites. It is effective for mild, uncomplicated contact eczemas. Where the skin is thickened and lichenified, referral is probably best so that consideration can be given to the prescription of more potent topical steroids.

Weeping lesions

Wet lesions may or may not be infected. Provided that the exudate is clear and watery, as occurs in some cases of eczema, the application of potassium permanganate soaks (see p 136) for about 15 minutes three times a day can sometimes produce good results. Patients with any purulent or unusual discharge should be referred.

Antifungal agents

The imidazoles, e.g. clotrimazole, miconazole and econazole, are effective topical antifungal agents and have largely superseded more traditional preparations such as Whitfield's ointment (benzoic acid and salicylic acid). They are effective against tinea cruris, tinea corporis and tinea pedis, as well as candidiasis. This broad spectrum of activity makes them particularly suitable for the treatment of intertriginous rashes, where the exact causative infective agent may not be clear. They may be used in a combination product with hydrocortisone where the rash is particularly irritant. Terbinafine cream is an equally effective treatment for tinea pedis and tinea cruris.

Tolnaftate is effective against tinea but has little activity against *Candida*.

Treatment for tinea and *Candida* infections must be continued for at least one week (and preferably longer) after symptoms have subsided to ensure complete eradication of the infection.

Potassium permanganate soaks are also a useful supplement in moist areas and where the skin is macerated, as in the toe webs in tinea pedis (see Figure 13.5).

Parasiticidal agents

Treatment of scabies

The scabies mite, *Sarcoptes scabiei*, burrows into the epidermis and leaves eggs and faeces behind it. Protein material in the faeces causes an allergic reaction in the skin. Patients should be advised that itching occurs several weeks after infection has occurred and may not disappear until a similar period after successful eradication of the mite. This information is important to convey, firstly, because symptomatic treatment with topical hydrocortisone or an oral antihistamine after using a scabicide may be appropriate and, secondly, because other individuals in close contact with the patient will also probably be already infected by the time the patient has symptoms. Infection is spread by close physical contact and hence it is necessary to treat all family members and sexual contacts at the same time.

As with head lice, it is both diplomatic and less stigmatising for pharmacists to use the word 'infection' rather than 'infestation' when discussing scabies with patients.

There is now a wide range of proprietary products for the treatment of scabies that has largely supplanted the traditional application of benzyl benzoate. The latter is irritant and this might also be a potential problem with alcoholic formulations. Thus, a non-alcoholic lotion of malathion or a cream containing permethrin may be the best recommendation.

Traditionally, patients were told to take a hot bath before applying a scabicide. This is deemed no longer necessary but the skin should be clean, cool and dry before application. The scabicide should be applied with cotton wool or a piece of sponge to the whole body, from the soles of the feet upwards but excluding the head and neck. Children under two years of age should not be treated without a referral first.

The scabicide penetrates the skin to kill the mite and eggs in the basal layer of the epidermis. Care should be taken to apply it between the fingers and toes and under the nails. Aqueous applications should be left on for 24 hours and alcoholic lotions for 12 hours. It is important to tell the patient that if the hands are inadvertently washed or immersed in water during this period, the scabicide should be re-applied.

It is not necessary to repeat the application. Because of residual itching, it may take up to three weeks before treatment can be deemed successful. If the patient is still symptomatic at this time, a referral to confirm the diagnosis is advisable.

Since the scabies mite cannot survive outside the human body, it is not necessary to make special arrangements about laundering or washing clothes and bed linen.

Treatment of body lice

Pubic lice are treated in a similar way to head lice with a lotion containing malathion or phenothrin (see Chapter 12). Where the eyelashes are affected, white soft paraffin can be smeared lightly over the lids and lashes twice daily for two or three weeks. This prevents the lice from respiring normally.

Body lice are treated in the same way as scabies (see above). The clothes and bedding should be washed.

Treatment of fleas

As already mentioned, the itchy skin lesions caused by flea bites can be treated with topical hydrocortisone or antihistamines, or oral antihistamines. However, attention to household furnishings is also necessary and it is useful to convey the lifecycle of the flea to patients to gain their co-operation and compliance in eradicating the problem. Cats and dogs harbour adult fleas in their coat. The fleas feed by sucking blood from the skin of their host and lay their eggs in the animal's fur. The eggs drop from the animal onto carpets, pet bedding, soft furnishings, etc. and hatch into larvae, which then migrate away from light under carpets, rugs and furniture. The larvae pupate before eventually hatching into the next generation of fleas, which search for a host (animal or human) to start the cycle again. Humans are usually bitten when fleas jump from their pets.

One of the available proprietary insecticidal products should be applied about the home to kill the adult fleas and prevent metamorphosis, with special attention to soft furnishings and areas under carpets and furniture. This should be accompanied by regular vacuuming, including under rugs and furniture, and cleaning of pet bedding. Finally, the pet itself should be treated by application of one of the proprietary insecticidal topical products, available from pet supply shops, on a regular basis to prevent re-infestation.

Sunscreens

Although at one time the efficacy of sunscreens was judged by their ability to protect against UVB light, the importance of UVA in the pathogenesis of skin ageing and skin cancer has resulted in a requirement to protect the skin from both UVA and UVB. Products should be chosen which have a high sun protection factor (SPF) for UVB and a high star rating for UVA. This is also important with respect to drug-induced photosensitivity (largely mediated through UVA) and polymorphic light eruption (mediated through UVA and UVB).

Wart solvents

So-called wart solvents generally contain high concentrations of salicylic acid, a keratolytic agent, which will reduce the size of the wart but not remove it. Although warts will usually resolve spontaneously within two years or so, they are cosmetically unacceptable to many patients. If a proprietary solvent does not achieve the desired effect, a referral should be made for removal by freezing.

 SUMMARY OF CONDITIONS PRODUCING TRUNK AND LIMB LESIONS

Allergic contact eczema

Allergic contact eczema produces an erythematous rash, often localised to the contact point with the causative agent. Common causes are nickel (metal jewellery, buckles and jean studs), leather (shoes and watchstraps) and dyes (clothing).

Atopic eczema

Atopic eczema is often associated with a personal or family history of atopy (eczema, asthma, hay fever or urticaria). It appears as a dry, often scaly, erythematous rash (see Figure 13.6). It is very itchy and evidence of this is apparent by visible scratch marks (excoriations) in some patients. It is the commonest form of eczema in babies from three months of age. Although atopic eczema often resolves in childhood, it can continue into adulthood. It is common on the face, and in skin flexures, as in the wrists, the crease of the elbows and behind the knees. In some instances it may be vesicular. If eczema becomes a chronic condition, it runs a fluctuating course. Between acute exacerbations the skin will become dry, leading to cracking, which can be painful.

Cancer

There are three main types of skin cancers. Basal cell carcinomas, the commonest type, are usually ulcerating (rodent ulcers), relatively slow growing and never metastasise. They are commonly seen on exposed skin. They arise from the basal cell layer of the skin or in hair follicles. Initially they may appear as a small, innocent-looking, isolated red papule but eventually they develop raised or rolled edges, giving the typical appearance of an ulcer – **refer**.

Squamous cell carcinoma is common on exposed sites such as the face and arms. It may present as a rapidly growing or a slowly growing nodule that does not resolve – **refer**.

A melanoma can be malignant if not checked early. It is derived from collections of pigment cells in the skin (moles). Moles are common on healthy skin and are normally harmless. However, damage, such as from excessive sunlight, can trigger a change in nature and in appearance. At this stage, a medical opinion should be sought. Any sudden increase in size or colour change, bleeding, ulceration, pain or irritation indicates the need to – **refer**.

Drug eruptions

Drug rashes can take many different forms but the most common types are macular and maculopapular rashes, urticaria and photosensitivity (Figure 13.10). The first two types may be widespread in their distribution or confined to small areas on the limbs. They typically appear about three to seven days after

(continued overleaf)

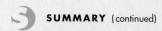

SUMMARY (continued)

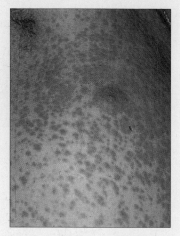

Figure 13.10   Antibiotic-induced rash. (Reproduced with permission from the Wellcome Trust Medical Photographic Library.)

starting the drug, but can occur much earlier (on the same day) if the patient has been exposed to the drug on a previous occasion. Drug-induced urticaria occurs relatively rapidly, within hours of administration. Photosensitive rashes induced by drugs resemble sunburn on light-exposed areas of the skin. They can be either rapid or slow in onset. Since the patient's doctor should be aware of such reactions to drugs – **refer**.

Irritant contact eczema
Irritant chemicals can cause trauma to the skin, resulting in an inflamed area at the point of contact. The condition is particularly common on the hands. Causes include oils, lubricants, inks, etc. at work, and detergents and washing-up liquids at home.

Intertrigo
Intertrigo describes a rash between occlusive or opposing folds of skin in which a moist warm environment favours the growth of *Candida* and tinea. It is more likely to occur in obese people, under the breasts in women, in the axilla and in the groin. The rash is often sore. It may respond to topical antifungal preparations, but severe cases may require referral.

Lichen planus
Lichen planus presents as small, flat-topped, pruritic, shiny papules, often with a purple colour initially (see Figure 13.7). White streaks may be seen on the surface. Sometimes its appearance may be similar to eczema. It affects the flexor aspects of the wrists, limbs and sometimes trunk and genitalia. Lesions may sometimes be seen in the mouth, where a white lace-like or streaky pattern can be seen on the buccal mucosa. The condition, which is of unknown aetiology, is self-limiting over several months. As it subsides, post-inflammatory hyperpigmentation imparts a brown colour to the lesions and in some cases this hyperpigmentation can appear without any obvious preceding inflammation. If the accompanying pruritus cannot be relieved with oral antihistamines, topical steroids may be required, in which case – **refer**.

Lichen simplex
Lichen simplex can be regarded as either a form of atopic eczema or a consequence of it. Intense itching causes skin thickening (lichenification; Figure 13.11). Scratching perpetuates the condition. If the pruritus is severe – **refer**.

Molluscum contagiosum
This condition occurs predominantly in children and is caused by a pox virus. Small, shiny, smooth, pearl- or flesh-coloured papules occur on the trunk, face or limbs (water warts; Figure 13.12). The lesions may be isolated or appear in groups and there are no symptoms. The condition eventually resolves and there is no satisfactory medical treatment.

→

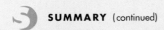

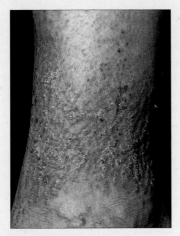

Figure 13.11 Lichen simplex. (Reproduced with permission from Glaxo Wellcome.)

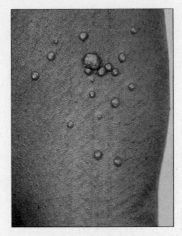

Figure 13.12 Molluscum contagiosum. (Reproduced with permission from the Wellcome Trust Medical Photographic Library.)

Polymorphic light eruption

Polymorphic light eruption is a reaction to sunlight and is often referred to as heat rash. It appears on light-exposed areas as erythema, with small macules, papules, or vesicles. It occurs in the spring and the summer. Sites frequently exposed to sunlight, such as the face and hands, are usually spared. The condition is most common in adolescents, particularly females, and appears within 24 hours of sun exposure. It is very itchy and is thought to be due to both UVA and UVB light. Sunscreens or a carefully developed suntan may help to protect the skin.

Pompholyx

Pompholyx is the name given to endogenous eczema (i.e. not contact eczema) of the hands (see Figure 13.1) or feet. Often the two sites are affected together. The condition starts as small vesicles (blisters), which may become bullae and burst. On the hands, the palms are usually affected. There is pruritus. Topical steroids are usually required – **refer**.

Prickly heat (miliaria)

Often referred to as sweat rash, prickly heat is an itchy rash occurring at sites of friction from clothing or following application of topical preparations that occlude the sweat ducts. Treatment involves avoiding tight clothing or offending materials.

Psoriasis

Psoriasis is a condition in which the rate of turnover of epidermal cells increases tenfold and the epidermis thickens. In its most common form, it presents as raised erythematous plaques covered with white or silvery scales (see Figure 13.3). The lesions vary in size and are often circular or oval patches. Common sites are the elbows, knees, scalp, sacrum, nails, intertriginous areas and sometimes the hands and feet. Psoriasis occurs most frequently in young adults and is usually a chronic condition that waxes and wanes in severity. There is often a strong family history in patients suffering from epilepsy. The condition is often

(continued overleaf)

SUMMARY (continued)

asymptomatic but there may be pruritus. The appearance of the rash and the exfoliation is the cause of much distress – **refer**.

Scabies

The scabies mite burrows into the skin and causes pruritus, leading to excoriation and sometimes secondary infection. Sometimes thin greyish burrows, about 0.5 cm long, can be seen. The skin erupts in small red papules (see Figure 13.2). The finger webs are classically affected first, and then the wrists, axillae, genitalia, buttocks and abdomen. The chest and upper back are rarely affected. Although the mite is found on the face and head, in adults the rash and pruritus do not occur at these sites. In young children and the elderly, however, the rash can involve the face (this condition is called crusted scabies).

Shingles

Shingles is caused by reactivation of the herpes zoster (chickenpox) virus which has lain dormant in a sensory root ganglion. The virus travels along the course of a nerve, producing the characteristic eruption of the skin and acute pain (see Figure 13.8). The rash may run from the back across the chest or around the abdomen. It classically is unilateral and finishes at the midline – **refer**.

Sunburn

Sunburn is a well-recognised acute, erythematous, inflammatory eruption occurring a few hours after excessive exposure to ultraviolet light. It is chiefly due to UVB; in severe cases, burns and blistering can occur. Sunburn may be accompanied by shivering, fever and nausea. Chronic exposure to sunlight can cause premature ageing of the skin and predispose to cancer – this is largely due to UVA.

Tinea cruris

Tinea (ringworm) infection of the groin area (Dhobie itch) is more common in men than women. It results in a scaly, erythematous, circular lesion, characterised by well-defined edges. The rash, which is symmetrical, appears to clear from the centre, is redder at the edges and spreads outwards. Pruritus is often present. The patient often als[...]

Tinea corporis

Ringworm infection of th[...]
isolated erythematous a[...]
cruris, the lesions have [...]
distinguishing tinea from[...]

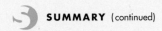

SUMMARY (continued)

Tinea pedis

Tinea infection of the foot (athlete's foot) appears in the toe clefts (classically between the fourth and fifth toes). It usually presents with itching, as a red, scaly eruption, and there may later be maceration and fissuring (see Figure 13.5). The condition can spread to other parts of the foot. Treatment is with topical antifungal agents.

Urticaria

An urticarial rash (Figure 13.13) has characteristic weals and erythema, and pruritus is usually present. It may occur on any part of the body. It is often part of an allergic reaction to drugs, foods, preservatives and colourants, although it is sometimes triggered by changes in temperature and fever. It generally only lasts about 24 hours and if mild can be treated with oral antihistamines. If the patient has considerable oedema, and especially if the oedema spreads to the eyelids and lips and occludes the upper airway (angioedema), the condition should be treated as a medical emergency. A tracheostomy can be lifesaving in such circumstances.

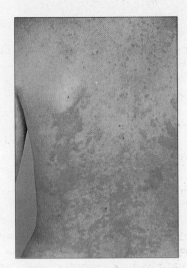

Figure 13.13   Urticaria. (Reproduced with permission from the Wellcome Trust Medical Photographic Library.)

Vitiligo

Vitiligo presents as patches of depigmented skin. There may be a hereditary link. The condition can affect the trunk and limbs as well as the face and is often distributed symmetrically on both sides of the body. It is generally symptomless and of no consequence, but care should be taken to protect lesions from an increased susceptibility to sunburn.

Warts

Warts are well-defined, benign epithelial outgrowths, associated with a virus. They are most common on the hands and fingers and the soles of the feet (verrucae). They may occur singly or in crops. Verrucae are painful when pressure is applied to them. Warts generally resolve spontaneously within two years. If they are particularly unsightly or unacceptable to the patient, they can be removed by freezing with liquid nitrogen. In such cases – **refer**.

WHEN TO REFER
Skin disorders: trunk and limbs

- Any skin rash, lesion or pruritus that does not respond to OTC management

Hands
- Erythema or vesicles on palms
- Inflamed, painful skin surrounding the nail
- Pitting of fingernails

Legs
- Erythematous rash or ulceration on the lower leg or ankles in an elderly person

Trunk
- Unilateral rash on the chest or abdomen that stops at the midline
- Photosensitive rash or urticaria in a patient taking prescribed medication
- Chickenpox in special cases such as in pregnancy or in a mother less than four weeks after childbirth, or if the patient either is prescribed steroids, is immunocompromised or is unwell
- Moles with two of the following characteristics:

    - Increasing in size
    - Change in shape or outline from regular to irregular
    - Change in colour or mixed colour in the same mole
    - Itching
    - Bleeding
    - Crusting
    - Inflammation

Genitalia
- Sores or blisters

Accompanying symptoms
- Skin lesions accompanied by: malaise, fever or swollen lymph glands
- Urticaria accompanied by swelling of eyelids, lips or difficulty in breathing – emergency referral
- Urticaria or photosensitivity rash in a patient taking prescribed medication

CASE STUDIES

Case 1

A young Asian man in his early 20s visits the pharmacy. He is a university student visiting his parents during the vacation, and is very anxious about an irritant rash. This is all over his trunk, but is particularly bad around his groin, axillae and wrists. He shows his wrists to the pharmacist.

'Could it be scabies?' he asks.

Even as he speaks he is scratching, suggesting he is probably right. The irritation is also much worse at night. The pharmacist examines the skin on the wrist, but can find no burrows. Aware this is often the case once the infection is established, the pharmacist turns to the hands and discovers a thin red line in the webs between several fingers. This, the pharmacist explains, is very characteristic. The young man is even more alarmed and has to be convinced that 'clean' people can get scabies, and that the infection must have started some weeks ago with a contact when he was at university. On dark skins it can be very difficult to find convincing signs, although in this case the patient's history means there can be no doubt.

The student leaves, a little relieved, with medication and instructions, although he calls by a week later complaining that the treatment has not worked. On checking, the pharmacist finds he has used the lotion entirely as directed but forgotten that the irritation may persist due to the debris remaining in the skin.

Case 2

A young woman asks for a prescription for head lice, for the children of a friend. She is understandably vague about their details but is sure they have lice and a quantity of lotion is supplied. She looks relieved.

Two weeks later she returns, requesting a further supply. The pharmacist is hesitant and suggests the children should be examined. She then admits the treatment is for her boyfriend, recently returned from a camping trip and listing among his souvenirs body lice. Embarrassment has caused them to use head lice lotion on both of them.

Ingenious, the pharmacist agrees, but there is a problem. The body louse lays eggs in clothing, not on the skin. The itchy rash is due to biting, but the insecticide must be applied to clothing too. It was cold when the boyfriend was away, and most of the party kept their clothes on in the tents at night, allowing the infection to develop.

An alternative treatment, the pharmacist recommends, is to wash in hot water all potentially affected clothing and bedding, for heat kills the lice. Ironing supplements this, and it is particularly useful to iron the seams, where the eggs are often laid, presumably out of the way and undisturbed.

Case 3

A young woman in her late teens has a very up-to-date problem. She recently has had a ring placed through the lower part of her umbilicus, as decoration. As she is wearing an outfit that does not quite meet in the middle, the pharmacist has little trouble inspecting it.

The skin around this ring is clearly inflamed, and the woman has been picking at it. As it was done only 10 days ago, it is tempting to assume this is only to be expected, and that using a topical anaesthetic for a short while will allow it to settle down. However, the skin is noticeably reddened, perhaps more than expected, and might be infected. In addition, she may have a previously unsuspected metal allergy, a view given credence when she discloses her difficulties in wearing rings and a wristwatch without 'getting sore'.

The pharmacist continues to ponder the problem, and the umbilicus, until the woman further offers that she has already tried her mother's topical steroid for a few days. It made things worse. An infection it is, and she is advised to telephone her doctor for help, leaving the pharmacy with advice on antiseptic care.

14

Childhood ailments

Many of the disorders of childhood that may present to pharmacists are dealt with in other chapters in this book. This chapter provides a summary of the more common disorders.

Skin disorders

Atopic eczema

Atopic eczema has a genetic link and the chance of developing the condition is increased if one or both parents suffer from eczema, hay fever or asthma. However, children can become atopic in the absence of an obvious family history.

Atopic eczema can begin as early as one month of age. It presents as red, itchy papules which may ooze and crust in the acute state but become dry and scaly when the condition becomes chronic. Common sites are the face and the flexures of the wrists, elbows and behind the knees. The condition causes intense irritation; scratching can lead to secondary infection. About 75 per cent of children outgrow their eczema by the early teenage years, but in a few cases the condition persists into adulthood as a chronic eczema.

Although many parents are adamant that a low allergen diet involving the exclusion of milk causes an improvement, the evidence for this is controversial. Babies and older children should not be given soya milk (soya feed) without the knowledge and approval of their doctor. Goat's milk can also be allergenic and is not a suitable alternative. Any kind of dietary manipulation requires the supervision of a doctor, dietitian or health visitor.

Mild cases of atopic eczema usually respond to emollients; an oral antihistamine will sometimes be useful at night. Soap should be avoided, as should detergents, including some bath additives. Wool fabrics and synthetic materials will also irritate the skin.

It is believed that breast-feeding provides immunoglobulin IgA, which combats allergens in the intestinal mucosa and so may protect against atopic eczema, but not all babies with atopic eczema will benefit in this respect.

Molluscum contagiosum

Molluscum contagiosum (water warts) is a common viral infection of the skin, which particularly affects infants and young children with eczema. It appears as small pearl-coloured drop-like papules, each having a small dimple in the centre. It can occur on the face but is more common on the limbs and trunk. The condition is not irritant and no treatment is necessary. It will resolve spontaneously after a few months. However, referral is necessary if the condition becomes infected or the child scratches the lesions.

Napkin dermatitis

Most babies develop napkin rash at some stage and it is a condition that often causes more distress to the parents than to the baby. Classically, it appears as a confluent red rash over the napkin area. In some cases it may take the form of papules or vesicles and there may be fissuring. The condition may be caused by a contact dermatitis from the ammonia released from the urine by faecal organisms and from other constituents of urine and faeces. It may be worsened by constant soaking of the skin in the napkin area. This contact dermatitis spares the intertriginous areas of skin (between skin folds) where there is no contact with the irritant urine and thus it can be distinguished from candidal infection, seborrhoeic eczema and psoriasis in which the intertriginous areas are affected.

Treatment includes more frequent nappy changes, gentle cleansing of the skin (no soap) and barrier creams. Whenever possible, the skin should be exposed by removing the nappy to allow drying and healing. At night-time, nappies can be placed like sheets under and above, but not around, the trunk, so facilitating some circulation of air.

Candidal napkin dermatitis

The wet, warm environment created under a nappy provides an ideal place for the growth of *Candida* and bacteria. Candidal infection of the napkin area causes a bright red eruption with pinpoint papules or pustules, covering all the skin, including intertriginous areas. It may be associated with oral candidiasis (thrush) and is a common sequela to antibiotic treatment.

Candidal infection should be suspected when a napkin rash fails to respond to simple symptomatic remedies. Treatment with topical imidazole creams should be tried for seven days; if there is no improvement, or if the rash spreads to the trunk, referral to the doctor should be considered.

Staphylococcal napkin dermatitis

If a nappy rash appears as a pustular rash, there may be bacterial infection. The pustules may rupture and produce scaling. If suspected, the patient should be referred for consideration of antibiotic treatment.

Seborrhoeic napkin dermatitis

This may appear as a red scaling eruption, especially in the intertriginous areas. Often the infant also has seborrhoeic eczema of the scalp (cradlecap), face, trunk and behind the ears.

Psoriatic napkin dermatitis

Psoriasis in the nappy area, which is rare, occurs initially as a red eruption. There may be some scaling, but not as much as is found in psoriasis that occurs elsewhere on the body. The condition may later spread to the trunk and limbs. Failure of nappy rash to resolve after several weeks of standard treatment may raise the possibility of napkin psoriasis and requires referral.

Seborrhoeic eczema

Seborrhoea may affect the intertriginous zones of the napkin area and spread to the trunk. It appears as a confluent papular red rash. On the scalp (cradlecap), forehead and behind the ears, seborrhoeic eczema appears with characteristic scaling. Cradlecap can be treated by softening the scales with olive oil or emulsifying ointment and then washing the scalp with a baby shampoo. Intertriginous seborrhoea may require topical steroids and referral is therefore indicated.

Head lice

Head lice are most commonly found in children, but adults can have them too. Head lice cannot jump and they can only spread by children touching heads, usually for some time. The head louse, *Pediculus capitis*, clings to hair with its claws and feeds on blood from the host's scalp (Figure 14.1). The louse has a lifecycle of about 20 days. Eggs are laid and attach themselves to hair shafts by means of a cement. After seven to 10 days, the eggs hatch and leave white, shiny egg cases (nits) on the hair (Figure 14.2). Within ten days, fully developed adult lice form.

Nowadays, most children's heads will be infected with as few as 10 to 20 lice. Such small numbers will be difficult to find with the naked eye and it is for this reason that inspection by the school nit nurse is a thing of the past. Infection may be asymptomatic in some children while in others there will be an itchy scalp, especially behind the ears. This itch can take a few weeks to develop after infection, since it is mani-

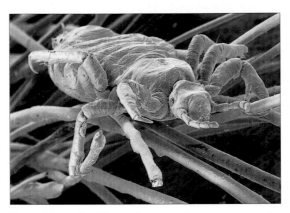

Figure 14.1 Head louse. Scanning electron micrograph of *Pediculus humanus capitis*, amongst hair. Acutal size is approx. 2–3 mm in length. The louse's three pairs of legs can be seen directly behind the head. (Reproduced with permission from Eye of Science/Science Photo Library.)

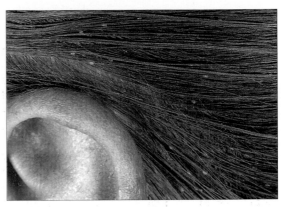

Figure 14.2 Head louse eggs (nits). (Reproduced with permission from Dr Chris Hale/Science Photo Library.)

festation of an allergic response to the lice, and by the same token the itch may persist for some time after successful eradication with insecticidal lotions.

Infection can only be reliably diagnosed when a louse is found and this can only be successfully done by detection combing.

Technique for detection combing

1. The hair should be wetted and dried to dampness to prevent lice moving when combed.
2. The hair is then combed with a normal comb to remove tangles.
3. The hair should then be combed using a plastic detection comb, starting at the roots and combing along the length of the hair. This process should be repeated several times.
4. The comb should be tapped out onto white paper to view any lice. Each louse is about the size of a pin head.
5. Any lice should be stuck to the paper with a piece of sellotape and taken to the pharmacy or nurse as proof of infection.
6. The comb should be washed under the tap.
7. Detection combing is best performed on all contacts and family members to diagnose who is infected. Family members should not be routinely treated unless lice have been detected.

Treatment of head lice

Treatment with insecticidal lotions should only be carried out when lice have been found by detection combing. If no lice have been seen, treatment is unnecessary. The use of insecticidal lotions as a preventative measure is not recommended.

OTC insecticides available include malathion, permethrin and phenothrin. All appear to be equally effective. Insecticidal shampoos have too short a contact time to be effective and thus lotions are to be recommended. They should be applied as follows.

1. Approximately 50 to 100 ml of insecticidal lotion will be needed per head, depending on the amount of hair.
2. The lotion must be applied to dry hair. The hair should be separated with the fingers to expose the scalp and then a small amount of lotion rubbed into the scalp until the scalp is wet. Special attention must be paid to the nape of the neck and behind the ears. For long hair the lotion should also be applied to the first one or two inches of the hair, which is the distance that the lice may move from the scalp.
3. It is advisable for the child to hold a towel over the face and eyes to avoid spillage while the parent applies the insecticide.
4. The hair should be allowed to dry naturally and the lotion left on, preferably overnight.
5. The lotion should be shampooed off the next day.

6. The application should be repeated after seven days if possible.
7. The hair can be inspected by detection combing a few days after the second application.
8. Where there is still evidence of infection (and only when the evidence is presented on a piece of paper beneath a square of sellotape) another insecticide may be used and friends and family also investigated for infection. If this fails, the patient is best referred to the doctor to consider a prescription for carbaryl.

The treatment of head lice requires a huge commitment from both patients and parents. Resistance to insecticides can occur, but the policy of rotation in a district is no longer justified. Most apparent treatment failures are due to poor technique, use of inadequate quantities of lotion, or forgetting that a persistent itch is not necessarily a sign of continued infection. Sometimes young lice, which have hatched from eggs after the first application, may be found after the first application of insecticide but they should not survive the second application.

The practice of 'bug busting' has been advocated, and is especially favoured by parents who consider chemical treatment undesirable. This technique involves wet combing of the hair with a detection comb until no more lice are found. Combing is done every three or four days for two weeks. If lice are found, the combing period is extended by another three to four days. There is, however, controversy about the effectiveness of this method.

Scabies

The intense itching of scabies is caused by an allergic reaction to the excreta of the mite *Sarcoptes scabei*, and it sometimes takes several weeks after infection before the pruritus begins. The pruritus is sudden in onset, severe and is worse at night. The rash is papular but not always obvious. The presence of a pruritic rash in other family members will provide a clue to its diagnosis. In infants and toddlers, the head and neck, trunk, wrists, palms, and soles and insteps of the feet are particularly affected.

Suitable scabicides for children are malathion and permethrin, but the latter is more suitable since it can be left on the skin for only eight hours, rather than 24 hours. Treatment should be applied to the whole body and details are given in Chapter 13. Children under two years of age should be referred for treatment under medical supervision and up to this age the face (up to and around the hairline), neck and ears should also be treated. If the hair is thin or fine, the scalp should be treated too. In older children, as in adults, with more dense hair, application of lotion is difficult and in any case infection is less likely on the scalp unless the child is immuno-compromised. In children over the age of two years, the treatment should be applied only on the body and not on the head and neck. Lotions containing permethrin should be left on for eight hours and care taken that children do not wash or put their hands in water during that time. The allergic reaction responsible for the pruritus may take two weeks to disappear, and during this time calamine lotion or crotamiton cream should be used to relieve symptoms.

Impetigo

Impetigo is caused by a staphylococcal or streptococcal infection of the skin. The condition is contagious, mostly affecting children of school age. The rash occurs most commonly on the face, chiefly around the nose and mouth, but sometimes also affecting the limbs. It begins as vesicles, which rupture and weep, with the affected skin becoming very red. The exudate then dries to form yellow-brown, sticky crusts. The skin is sore and scratching the lesions can cause the infection to spread to other sites. The condition is contagious and children should be kept from school until the lesions have dried up (usually only a few days).

Referral is necessary for topical or systemic antibiotic therapy.

Measles

Measles has become uncommon nowadays because of widespread immunisation. The virus is spread by droplet infection from the respiratory tract, and the incubation period (time between exposure and symptoms) is seven to 14 days. The condition begins with a fever and symptoms of an upper respiratory tract infection. Conjunctivitis and small red spots on the buccal mucosa of the mouth will often be present (Figure 14.3). After about four to five days, the rash appears and is blotchy and flat, starting on the face and then spreading down to the trunk and limbs. It lasts about seven days.

The child should be kept away from school for a minimum of seven days from the appearance of the rash.

Children who have been vaccinated may still have measles in a mild form. Standard treatment includes paracetamol for fever, and promethazine syrup if there is pruritus.

Chickenpox

Chickenpox is now the most common infectious disease of childhood. It spreads readily among school and family contacts, either by droplet infection from the respiratory tract or by contact with the vesicular exudate. The incubation period is between 10 and 24 days. Children may catch chickenpox from an adult with shingles, but not vice versa. The child should be excluded from school until the rash is dry and crusted, with all vesicles gone. Viral particles can be isolated from the vesicle fluid, increasing the infectivity. This usually takes at least one week from onset.

The chickenpox rash appears as characteristic tiny vesicles (small blisters) surrounded by reddened areas, mainly on the trunk rather than the face and limbs (Figure 14.4); it may appear also on the scalp. The rash develops over two to five days and the vesicles eventually burst and form crusts or scabs, which disappear after about 10 days. Early on, both forms of the rash will be simultaneously found on the skin, i.e. vesicles and scabs.

The condition is very irritant but patients should be persuaded not to scratch the lesions since this may cause scarring and also releases the virus from the vesicles.

Complications are rare in children, although immunocompromised patients must be referred to the doctor. Standard treatment is with calamine lotion and oral antihistamines.

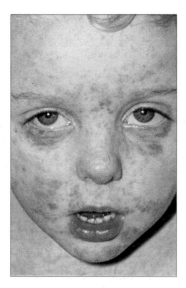

Figure 14.3 Measles. (Reproduced with permission from the Wellcome Trust Medical Photographic Library.)

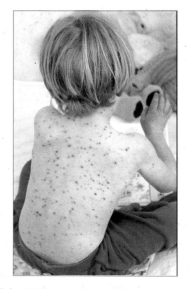

Figure 14.4 Chickenpox. (Reproduced with permission from Mark Clarke/Science Photo Library.)

Gastrointestinal

Oral candidiasis

Oral candidiasis (thrush) commonly occurs in babies as white patches on the tongue and buccal mucosa. It may be treated with oral antifungal gels. If it follows a course of antibiotics or there is evidence of candidal infection of skin in the napkin area, referral is needed for treatment with an oral agent, such as nystatin, to eradicate the infection from the gut.

Vomiting and diarrhoea

Vomiting and diarrhoea, either together or alone, are usually mild, benign symptoms in babies and older children.

Gastroenteritis, in a mild or severe form, is more common in bottle-fed than breast-fed infants. Mild or short episodes will resolve spontaneously, as in adults. However, symptoms lasting more than 24 hours in babies less than six months old or more than 48 hours in children under two years should be referred if there is no sign of improvement.

The major complication of vomiting or diarrhoea is dehydration, resulting in electrolyte and water imbalance. This can lead to severe illness. It would be extremely rare for a child to become significantly dehydrated within the time span referred to above without appearing obviously ill and in need of referral. However, electrolyte replacement mixtures are available and may be recommended by pharmacists.

Some babies have a habit of bringing up small amounts of milk after a feed (posseting). Provided that weight gain is normal, this is of no significance and the parents can be reassured.

Pyloric stenosis

Pyloric stenosis is a congenital defect of the pyloric sphincter in the stomach which prevents some of the ingested food passing into the duodenum, with the result that it is vomited.

The condition can become symptomatic within a few weeks of birth. It may be differentiated from the more common causes of infantile vomiting (such as virus infections) by the projectile nature of the vomiting. Large quantities are ejected with considerable force and travel some distance from the patient. Constipation frequently accompanies pyloric stenosis and in severe cases there may be dehydration. If suspected, the baby should be referred.

Colic

A baby that cries after a feed has usually been underfed or has swallowed an excessive amount of air. In bottle feeding, the latter may be caused by the baby sucking too hard on a teat with a small hole or a gulping action while trying to keep pace with the rapid flow of milk from a teat with a large hole. Large quantities of air cause distension of the stomach. If changing the size of the hole in the teat does not resolve the problem, a trial of a preparation containing simethicone may be warranted.

Infantile colic (evening or three months' colic) classically appears between two weeks and four months of age. It is characterised by rhythmical bouts of screaming, each lasting a few minutes, in an otherwise thriving baby. If the crying does not abate when the mother picks up the baby (as would be the case if a baby is lonely, cold or has a wet napkin), then it is possible that gastric or intestinal spasm is causing pain. If crying persists for several hours, or if the baby is vomiting, then it is wise to refer.

There is a paucity of effective remedies for colic, but preparations containing simethicone may be useful. Mothers should be reassured that the condition will resolve eventually.

Food allergy or intolerance

True food allergy occurs in early childhood, but is relatively rare. It presents as an immediate anaphylactic reaction to food proteins, mediated by immunoglobulin IgE antibodies and is a medical emergency. Typical symptoms are urticaria, bronchospasm and angioedema (swelling of the face and throat). Typical causative agents are cow's milk and eggs, but many children grow out of these allergies. Allergies to nuts, though rare, are usually lifelong and can be fatal.

Non-immunological reactions to food are more common than true food allergy, but they are nevertheless referred to as food allergy by the lay person. Food allergy can only be diagnosed by skinprick tests or serum detection of IgE by a hospital specialist. Food intolerance may be due to a true chemical or physical reaction to food, but there are often psychological overtones. The most common symptom is vomiting. Exclusion diets can be used to identify the offending food and these are best performed under the supervision of either a dietitian or specialist.

Threadworm

Threadworm infestation characteristically causes severe perianal pruritus and sometimes pain, especially at night, which is when the female worms migrate to the anus to lay their eggs. Treatment is with piperazine [two doses 14 days apart for the powder and daily for seven days (repeated after one week if necessary) for the elixir] or mebendazole (single dose).

All family members should be treated and hygiene measures emphasised, such as washing the hands thoroughly after visiting the toilet.

Feeding difficulties

Breast feeding

Breast milk has many advantages over artificial milks and is the milk of choice.

Feeding difficulties are best dealt with, in the majority of cases, by advising the mother to seek the advice of her health visitor. Although not usually serious, feeding problems should not be trivialised and sympathy and appropriate referral should be the rule.

Overfeeding is unusual, but underfeeding is more common and is usually detected by crying at the end of, or between, feeds. For breast-

fed babies who cry because of underfeeding, the practice of using complementary bottle feeding has been superseded by the use of cup feeding. Breast-fed babies will often not suck on a bottle teat but the sucking reflex is simulated when milk (artificial or expressed) is offered instead via a baby cup. Oversupply in relation to demand by the baby may cause some women to develop engorged, painful breasts. In such cases, a breast pump should not be used to remove milk since this will only stimulate the breasts to produce more. The health visitor will be able to recommend appropriate measures, such as a reduction in the mother's fluid intake.

Where a breast pump is used to express milk for use at a later date, breast milk can be stored safely either in a refrigerator for 24 hours (or 72 hours if the temperature is kept below 4°C) or frozen for up to three months.

Breast-fed babies pass stools that are looser and more frequent than bottle-fed babies. However, if breast-fed babies develop diarrhoea, it is important that breast feeding should continue in addition to oral rehydration fluids.

Mothers sometimes develop cracked or sore nipples whilst breast feeding and such cases should be referred to the health visitor for advice, since sometimes technique or positioning of the baby at the breast may be responsible.

Breast pads can be used to absorb any leakage of milk from the breasts between feeds. Such leakage is quite normal, but again mothers should be encouraged to talk to the health visitor for reassurance and advice.

Bottle feeding

It is necessary to stress to mothers the importance of following exactly the manufacturer's instructions for preparing formula-milk feeds. Too much powder can result in an excess of electrolytes and a disturbance of fluid balance, with potentially serious consequences. The size of the hole in the bottle teat may be a problem, as mentioned above.

The sugar content of different brands of milk varies and this can affect bowel action. Too little sugar results in dry, hard stools and too much in large quantities of loose stools and diarrhoea.

Because of various nutritional deficiencies, cow's milk is inappropriate as a main drink for infants under 12 months, as is soya milk (unless on medical advice) and unmodified goat's milk, both of which are often recommended for children with milk allergies.

Skimmed milk should not be given to children below five years of age, since it lacks fat, a valuable energy source, and could lead to deficiency of the fat-soluble vitamins (A, D, E and K). Semi-skimmed milk may be given to children between two and five years.

Respiratory tract

Infections

Respiratory tract infections can cause distress to babies and young children out of proportion to the severity of the infection because of the narrow airway. Usually no treatment is necessary, although symptomatic relief is often given by inhalant balms or capsules. These should not be put on a baby's skin and generally are not recommended in infants under three months. When used, the inhalant should be dabbed on a handkerchief and placed out of reach, since a high concentration of volatile oils close to the airways has been thought to induce reflex apnoea in a few cases.

If a baby stops feeding, is febrile or appears generally unwell or different from normal, then a referral should be made.

Benign coughs are often worse at night, but persistent night-time coughs, wheezing or breathlessness are signals for referral to exclude such conditions as asthma.

Some children between the ages of four and eight years develop a chronic catarrhal syndrome comprising recurrent colds, coughs and earache. Provided that other possible conditions have been excluded and a doctor seen previously, the parents require only reassurance that no treatment is necessary, and that the condition will resolve eventually.

Tonsillitis

A sore throat is often thought by parents to be tonsillitis, but this is rarely the case. The tonsils normally appear as oval, fleshy red glands at either side of the back of the throat. White (pus-filled) patches speckled on the surface of the tonsils indicates acute tonsillitis and requires referral to the doctor. There is otherwise no need for referral unless the child appears ill in any other way, such as with feverishness, headache or earache.

In children, especially adolescents, a sore throat that persists for longer than one week or is recurrent and follows a week or two of malaise, or is accompanied by enlarged cervical lymph nodes, requires referral to exclude complications such as glandular fever.

Croup

Croup refers to the cough associated with partial airways obstruction in the larynx. It is more common at night and in babies and young children. The breathing is noisy and there is a characteristic high-pitched wheezing, which can be heard during the cough on expiration. The child will be distressed and appear ill. Croup is caused by oedema and narrowing of the airway resulting from inflammation around the larynx, epiglottis and vocal cords. It is rare and requires instant medical referral.

Whooping cough

Although most children are vaccinated against whooping cough, the disease can still occur in a mild form. It may present as a dry, irritating cough leading to continuous bouts of coughing, terminated by the characteristic whooping noise when the child takes a long, deep inspiration. In its mild presentation, the whoop may be absent. If a cough continues for 10 days, without improvement, and is accompanied by general malaise, anorexia or weight loss, the patient should be referred.

Teething

The eruption of the first teeth can be accompanied by a syndrome of inflamed painful gums, fever and irritability, and often the symptoms of a mild upper respiratory tract infection. Mothers will usually have diagnosed the problem themselves. Treatment is with paracetamol for the fever and pain, and this is generally more effective than a teething gel.

Earache

Ear pain in children always warrants referral to determine whether there is an infection (otitis media) and to consider appropriate treatment. Not all doctors will automatically prescribe antibiotics and it may be wise to advise parents that they need to seek the doctor's opinion about the condition but not necessarily to expect a prescription for antibiotics.

Headache

After a fall or head injury, children should be observed over the next 24 hours for signs of concussion such as drowsiness, lack of co-ordination, nausea or vomiting. Any of these symptoms require referral.

Children will suffer headaches that are of short duration, of no consequence and responsive to paracetamol, in the same way as adults. However, severe or recurrent headaches, those with other symptoms such as visual disturbances and those that are ended by vomiting should be referred for exclusion of conditions such as migraine.

Meningitis is an inflammation of the membranes enveloping the brain and spinal cord. The cardinal symptoms are headache (although some children will be too young to verbalise this), neck or back stiffness, fever, photophobia, nausea and vomiting, irritability or drowsiness. These symptoms are non-specific and a high index of suspicion is necessary. Meningitis usually occurs secondarily to bacterial infection elsewhere, following upper respiratory infection, or viral infection, including mumps and measles. The potentially rapidly fatal form is caused by a meningococcus. This form is associated with a purple purpuric rash (haemorrhagic, bruise-like spots of varying sizes) and is characterised by its extremely fast onset and rapid deterioration of the patient. While all epidemics have to start somewhere, meningococcal meningitis is rare, particularly in the absence of other locally reported cases. However, the seriousness of the diagnosis should leave it as a possibility in every pharmacist's mind.

CASE STUDIES

Case 1

Over the course of a few days a pharmacist in a busy urban pharmacy notices a sudden increase in the requests for head lice shampoo. The pharmacist's first response is to ask clients whether living lice have actually been isolated, and advise on how to identify them if necessary. For the few people that return after positive detection, a suitable lotion is recommended, rather than the shampoo.

The pharmacist remembers one woman in particular. She returns to the shop and demands to speak 'in the utmost confidence'. The whole of her son's class at school, it transpires, has been advised to seek treatment from their doctor or pharmacist after what is described as an outbreak of head lice. But, she insists, her son is very clean, showers daily, and the whole family is outraged by the notion he has lice. The school kitchens, she says, are not so well looked after and are clearly the source of the infection. The pharmacist attempts to reassure her: lice live on clean, healthy hair, not on food. Infection among school friends is rare, close head-to-head contact being the prerequisite. She reluctantly leaves with sufficient treatment.

No more is heard until she returns two months later, her son in tow and sporting a head louse, entombed in a fold of sticky tape; the living, or in this case dead, proof of her assertions. The pharmacist accepts there has been re-infection but disputes the origin. Some time is spent revisiting the boy's social contacts, and his grandmother, with whom he often has tea on his way home from school, emerges as a possibility. She is added to the list of suspects to be examined.

A further week passes before the grandmother herself appears. She has indeed found lice, but cannot think how they got there. Surely the infection must be the other way round, from her grandson to her. Interestingly she has no symptoms, and only a few lice. The pharmacist explains gently that tolerance to the irritation occurs with time, leaving an asymptomatic carrier state from which others may be infected. They both agree to keep this discovery too in the utmost confidence.

Case 2

A single woman, in her late 20s, is a frequent visitor to the pharmacy. She has two young children and life has clearly not been easy for her after the break-up of her marriage and the hostility she has suffered from her ex-husband during and after the breakup.

Both children suffer from frequent minor illnesses, and their prescription medicines are often supplemented with OTC remedies, particularly for colds and persistent coughs. More recently she has been buying vitamin supplements, which she says her doctor has told her may boost their immunity against infection. These dietary supplements become more frequent with time, especially for her youngest child, now aged four. Additional requests are made for iron and general tonics, which are referred back to her doctor. One day she states firmly that she wants to purchase a large quantity of a soya milk substitute, again on her doctor's advice.

The pharmacist offers to speak to her doctor, an offer made before but never accepted. Now the pharmacist feels this consultation is essential. The mother admits that the soya milk substitute is not her doctor's idea, but the result of extensive reading of magazines and the advice of friends. The conclusion reached is that her four-year-old has developed widespread food allergies, as he has become a very poor eater and is pale and tired. He lives on chips, biscuits and snacks. He still suffers frequent colds and has seen his doctor, who treats the infections when appropriate but dismisses the idea of allergy. The pharmacist sympathises with the mother's concerns, agrees there is clearly a problem and discusses it in some detail. Food allergy is uncommon, although food intolerance is more likely. Food phobia is perhaps most likely, and it is vital to find out which it is since the treatment will be different for each.

→

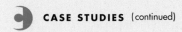 **CASE STUDIES** (continued)

Fortunately the practice health visitor, who knows the family well, is a customer with her own children and, with permission, is alerted to the problem. Her concerns in turn reach the doctor, and referral is arranged to a paediatrician. Investigations show normal immunoglobulins but a mild nutritional anaemia. The child is put on both iron and vitamin supplements, this time prescribed, and receives support and dietary re-education. The whole family have entered a behavioural therapy class and are coming to terms with the trauma they have survived, but perhaps not yet recovered from.

Case 3

A mother and her 10-year-old son seek the pharmacist's advice. Last Christmas was ruined by a dose of 'the flu', and now his passion for football is under similar threat. Deep into the season, he has missed so much time that he fears being dropped from the local team. The doctor cannot help, having checked him and passed him fit, except for a run of colds, which in fairness are afflicting many of his friends and team mates.

The pharmacist takes a detailed symptomatic history, and considers the best medicine that can be advised while they speculate on the cup final.

Things take a turn for the worst when the boy misses not only three consecutive training sessions but quite a lot of school. His mother again consults the pharmacist, who again takes a careful history. The colds are at their worst when out playing football, and when journeying down a busy road to and from school. The pharmacist finally asks the question, 'Do his eyes ever sting or water?'

It transpires that although the unfortunate lad certainly suffered a series of upper respiratory infections during the winter, he has passed now into his first year of hay fever, although this too is a misnomer. His allergens include the increasingly important vehicle emissions and the pollens from the trees that surround the playing field, which are active some weeks before the grass itself.

15

Foot disorders

Assessing symptoms

Site or location

Ascertaining the precise location of a problem in the foot is probably the most useful exercise in the identification of its cause (Figure 15.1).

Corns, the callosities of thickened skin formed by repeated but minor friction, will invariably arise over prominent sites such as the dorsal surface of interphalangeal joints of the toes (see Figure 15.4), the prominence of the heel bone (calcaneum), and under the metatarsal heads on the ball of the foot (see Figure 15.3).

Verrucae, which can produce reactive hard pads of thickened skin around them and appear similar to corns, are commonly found on the underside of the foot (see Figure 15.6).

A painful inflammation of the metatarsophalangeal joint of the great toe (the hallux) may be caused by gout or a bunion. A bunion is a swelling caused by a lateral displacement of this joint (see Figure 15.2).

Fungal infections of the feet usually arise in the clefts between the toes. The skin here is warm, often moist, and may be cracked, allowing a portal of entry to the organisms. A close examination of these clefts should reveal softening and inflammation of the skin, at least in a minor form, with characteristic peeling of its outer layers. In contrast, eczema affecting the feet is usually found on the flat surfaces, sparing the toe clefts, where the irritants often responsible cannot penetrate.

On the sole of the foot, plantar fasciitis, an inflammation of the longitudinal arch ligament, causes pain that runs forwards from the heel on weight bearing. This condition can be distin-guished from metatarsalgia, in which the pain is felt under one or more of the metatarsal heads, or transversely across several of them.

The pain from a twisted ankle is felt along the line of either the medial or lateral ligaments of the joint, depending on the direction of the injury. Lateral twists are more common, and may be confirmed by palpating the ligament, which stretches in a straight line from the bony extremity at the distal end of the tibia diagonally down to the end of the fifth metatarsal, the bony point approximately two-thirds of the way back on the side of the foot (see Figure 15.1). Acute tenderness will be found somewhere on this line; if, however, the maximum response is on either of the bones, a fracture may be suspected.

Pain and inflammation, with or without infection, along the lateral sides of a toenail, typically of the great toe, suggests an ingrowing toenail. In this condition, a spicule of nail is trapped by and later grows into the nail fold, i.e. the ridge between the side of the toe and the nail bed.

Pain in the heel from bursitis is discussed in Chapter 11.

Severity

Patients with severe pain in the foot or ankle will be unable to walk easily and thus will comparatively rarely present to the pharmacist. Differentiation should be made between pain that is constant and that brought about or greatly aggravated by weight bearing. A constant pain around the first metatarsophalangeal joint, at the base of the great toe, may be an attack of gout, while a similar distribution of pain present all the

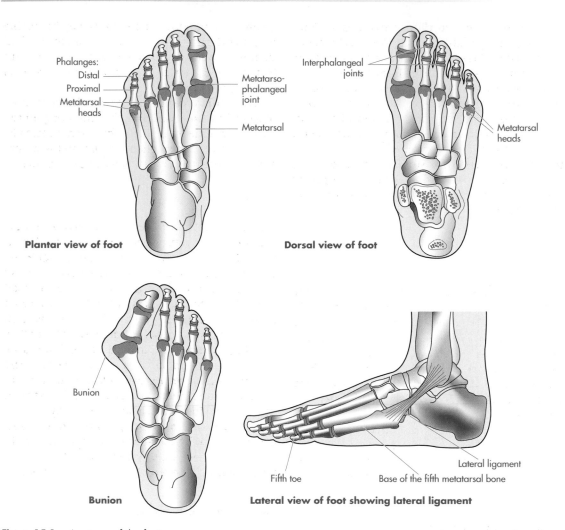

Plantar view of foot

Phalanges:
Distal
Proximal
Metatarsal heads

Metatarso-phalangeal joint

Metatarsal

Dorsal view of foot

Interphalangeal joints

Metatarsal heads

Bunion

Bunion

Lateral view of foot showing lateral ligament

Lateral ligament

Base of the fifth metatarsal bone

Fifth toe

Figure 15.1   Anatomy of the foot.

time but made worse on walking is more descriptive of an inflamed bunion (hallux valgus).

The conditions more frequently brought to the attention of the pharmacist will be less acute and may be pain free. Foot infections, often fungal or viral in nature, cause irritation rather than frank pain; minor deformities, with their resulting corns and calluses, usually cause most pain on walking.

Verrucae, like corns, are usually painless until pressure is applied on walking.

Duration

It is convenient to consider most conditions of the feet as either of short duration (acute) or long lasting (chronic). Into the former category will come those based on, or aggravated by, trauma, such as strains, sprains and friction injuries, as well as the potentially more serious thromboembolic problems and bony injuries. Repeated but low-grade trauma to the bony prominences of the feet in the elderly or those with ill-fitting footwear will result in a callus or corn; acute trauma to these areas, arising from sporting pursuits, after walking long distances or when fashion takes precedence over practicality, will result in a simple but painful blister.

For the most part, pharmacists will be asked for advice on chronic conditions. Athlete's foot, a fungal infection, can be present for months, if not years, and is often recurrent, even after treatment.

Verrucae that are not treated, as well as some that are, can persist for similar periods of time, as can minor but distressing orthopaedic conditions, including plantar fasciitis and metatarsalgia.

Onset

The speed of onset can give clues to the aetiology of many foot problems. Obviously, a fracture will be immediately painful after the causative injury. A severe ligamentous strain can produce as much pain, swelling and disability as a fracture but may have a slower onset. This means, for example, that a sportsman may return to the field after the injury, only later feeling the full effect of the insult.

Thromboses of either the arterial or venous systems of the foot or leg are extremely rare, but a sudden unexplained and severe pain should trigger consideration of this possibility.

Accompanying symptoms

Pain and inflammation

The predominant symptom accompanying an injury to the foot is pain. This is usually felt maximally at the point of damage, although sometimes the pain may radiate to where the tissues are under greatest strain or to the weight-bearing point of contact. Thus, an inflamed plantar fasciitis at the calcaneum may produce pain in the longitudinal arch of the foot, although when examined the tenderness will be further back.

The inflammatory exudate associated with injury produces swelling, and rupture of blood vessels adds discoloration. Because the foot is largely comprised of muscles and tendons held in lubricating sheaths, supported by less elastic ligaments and bones, these fluids may be unable to expand freely where they originate, or find their way to the subcutaneous spaces locally, and instead track down the sheaths to appear as swelling or bruising.

With inflammation, areas of the foot may become hot and red. During an attack of gout the area around the base of the great toe becomes visibly reddened and swollen, and hot to the touch, as well as painful. This is rarely true of trauma.

Infection

Infections of the feet must be regarded with some caution. While minor tineal infections are irritating but of no serious significance, bacterial infections can spread rapidly and cause both local and systemic effects. Through an abrasion or small laceration, the organisms enter the foot and an ascending cellulitis begins. The area is hot, painful and swollen. The same sheaths that allow tracking of extracellular fluids are colonised by the bacteria, with rapid upward spread. These cramped structures are particularly vulnerable to damage and subsequent scarring, and treatment must be provided quickly and vigorously.

Verrucae can be distinguished from corns under the foot by the appearance of black dots in their core. These are blood vessels in the dermis, visible when the overlying skin is rubbed off.

Coldness and discoloration

Some conditions can produce areas of cold in the feet. Chilblains start as white, cold, avascular patches of skin before developing into the typical hot, red, flame-shaped areas, usually on or around the toes. A potentially more serious and generalised embarrassment of the arterial circulation is seen in Raynaud's phenomenon, a constitutional tendency to vasoconstriction that causes painful cold feet, usually with similar signs of vasoconstriction elsewhere, typically in the fingers.

Thromboses of blood vessels within, or supplying, the foot will produce marked and severe symptoms. Arterial blockage results in pain and in a loss of blood supply, leaving the foot cold and white, while a venous thrombosis causes congestion, the painful foot being swollen and blue or even black in colour. Such acute events are rare. More chronic disruption of the circulation is common. Atherosclerosis will produce a pale and cold extremity; if unchecked, this may progress to an area of local gangrene, the skin turning blue and finally black, while the affected part (usually a toe) withers and dies. Such lesions should be suspected in smokers, patients with diabetes, those with other forms of arterial disease and with increasing age.

Rashes

Rashes that affect the feet can similarly affect other parts of the body. Fungal infections may occur as part of more widespread disease, with similar lesions in other areas, especially the groin.

Eczema on the feet, which is often aggravated by contact irritants in footwear, may be reflected in more generalised eczema. In chronic forms, especially on the sole of the foot, the condition produces hyperkeratosis and the patient will complain of hard skin. If the skin is not hydrated, it may crack and cause pain, especially where pressure is applied on walking, such as on the heel and the metatarsal heads.

Arthritis

Bunions are common in patients with rheumatoid arthritis, as are calluses. The latter are often caused by deformity of the joint alignment such that the metatarsophalangeal joints become subluxed and the patient walks on the metatarsal heads.

Aggravating factors

Ill-fitting shoes can cause or aggravate a number of foot problems, particularly bunions and corns. Sport shoes, including trainers, tend to be worn a size too small. There should be a half-inch gap between the end of the big toe and the edge of the training shoe. Patients who suffer hyperhydrosis (excessive perspiration) or bromhidrosis (odorous perspiration due to bacterial breakdown of sweat) and wear training shoes should be encouraged to wear two pairs on alternate days to allow them to dry out.

Incorrect nail cutting may lead to ingrowing toenails. This happens when the nail is cut too short or tapered at the sides, instead of being trimmed straight across.

Incidence and recurrence

Verrucae are extremely common in children, although by no means restricted to them. It is assumed that one method of spread is by barefoot contact, and infected school children are often banned from physical training and swimming, or condemned to wear unsightly occlusive rubber socks. There is in fact little evidence for this type of spread, and experiments allowing free contact have shown little consequent rise in the incidence of these infections. Some authorities believe that the child's immunological status and their ability to resist infection are more important in both the acquisition and the duration of the infection.

Verrucae may be difficult to differentiate from corns – the latter are more common in middle age and beyond, whereas verrucae are seldom seen in this age group.

Fungal infections have a tendency to recur, even after apparently adequate treatment. Again, resistance to the infection may be a factor. Also, these organisms have the ability to spore and to lie dormant for long periods of time; once established, even enthusiastic and protracted treatment may leave sufficient spores to await a more favourable opportunity.

Management

Injuries

Bandages and padding materials of foam or felt are useful in supporting strains, sprains and sporting injuries during recovery and in limiting the movement of affected parts. This will reduce pain, rest damaged tissues, speed recovery and help prevent further injury. Even if used improperly, such products will do little harm. Some, however, such as arch supports and metatarsal pads, although efficacious, may not immediately be comfortable to use.

Stubbing the foot against an unforgiving surface, or dropping a heavy weight on the toes, can give rise to swollen, bruised and very tender toes, which may even be fractured. If there is no apparent deformity, and no question of injury to the metatarsal bones, an X-ray of the foot is of doubtful value as it will not influence the management. The patient can be advised to place a support of gauze or something similar between the toes to preserve the space and stop them rubbing, and then to bind the injured toe to the next largest one.

Corns and verrucae

Many OTC preparations are available for the treatment of corns and verrucae, and are often purchased without advice. However, impregnated corn plasters, corn pastes and verruca treatments used indiscriminately or over a protracted period can be harmful and it might be wise to situate them close to the pharmacy counter so as to be in a position to offer advice to potential purchasers.

Most medicated corn and callus plasters contain not less than 40 per cent salicylic acid, in a variety of bases, and verruca dressings contain a minimum of 10 per cent salicylic acid. Other liquid and ointment formulations contain at least 10 per cent salicylic acid. The surrounding normal skin should be protected. Verrucae may be soaked in a formalin solution for 10 to 15 minutes but this can cause irritation of soft skin, such as between the toes.

All OTC packs carry health warnings for those with diabetes – it should be remembered, however, that one complication of diabetes is a deterioration in vision.

Some products carry a warning against use in those with circulation problems and an age range for treatment of between 16 and 50 years. However, an assessment of vascular efficiency is probably beyond most people. The results of over-liberal application can be quite severe, especially in those with impaired circulation. Treatment can produce pain and inflammation or, in more severe cases, tissue maceration and occasionally ulceration.

It would be worth considering medical referral before the use of high-strength salicylic acid preparations in the elderly or those taking certain other medication, such as anticoagulants or oral steroids, in whom the consequences of ulceration could be particularly severe.

Fungal infections

Tinea infections can be treated effectively with terbinafine or imidazole creams, such as clotrimazole, miconazole and econazole. The user should be advised to continue administration until several days after all traces of the infection have gone. Benzoic acid ointment is also effective, although cosmetically less acceptable. The undecenoates are probably less effective, and have largely been superseded.

More rarely, candidal infection may be found in the toe clefts, especially in the elderly, in patients with diabetes and in the immunocompromised. Again, imidazole creams are effective. Dusting the toe clefts with antifungal powders is useful in addition to, but not instead of, application of cream. If fungal infection cannot be excluded, topical hydrocortisone preparations are contraindicated unless in combination with an antifungal agent.

Ingrowing toenails

Ingrowing toenails are best treated by doctors or chiropodists. The offending spike of nail needs to be resected carefully under local anaesthetic, shaping the nail to prevent a recurrence.

SUMMARY OF CONDITIONS PRODUCING FOOT DISORDERS

Bunion
A bunion (hallux valgus) is a lateral displacement of the first metatarsophalangeal joint, causing a swelling of the bursa that lies above it (Figure 15.2). It results in a marked increase in the prominence at the base of the toe, and a compensatory inturning of the toe itself, with bunching and compression of the other toes. Tight shoes and high heels aggravate it. If severe or disabling – **refer**.

Calluses
A callus is a hardening or thickening of the skin over joints and areas of weight bearing and friction (Figure 15.3). It is similar in appearance to a corn, but larger in size.

Cellulitis
Cellulitis is an infection of the subcutaneous or deeper tissues, often streptococcal in origin. It may spread rapidly and needs an early medical assessment and treatment – **refer**.

Chilblains
Chilblains are produced by a localised area of ischaemia. They are induced by cold and are common when the peripheral circulation is embarrassed. The affected area of skin is initially white, later becoming red and finally bluish. Chilblains are often multiple and painful. Susceptible patients should be advised to dress warmly. Serious cases should be referred.

Corns
Corns are hardened areas of skin (Figure 15.4), produced in response to trauma. They occur when the skin over bony prominences is irritated by ill-fitting footwear or deformities of the feet, such as hammer toes or bunions.

Fungal infections
Athlete's foot is caused by tineal infection, and is commonly seen as maceration between the toes. From this site, the infection may spread to adjacent parts of the foot and can cause considerable irritation. It can usually be treated with OTC preparations. If the diagnosis is in doubt or the toenail is affected – **refer**.

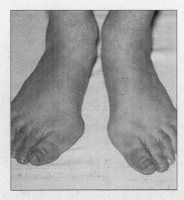

Figure 15.2   Bunions. (Reproduced with permission from the Wellcome Trust Medical Photographic Library.)

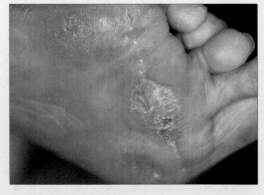

Figure 15.3   Callus. (Reproduced with permission from the Wellcome Trust Medical Photographic Library.)

→

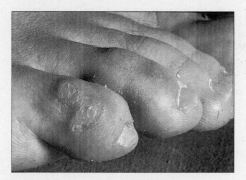

Figure 15.4   Corn. (Reproduced with permission from the Wellcome Trust Medical Photographic Library.)

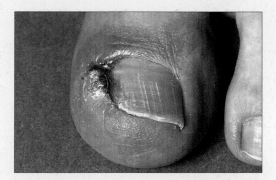

Figure 15.5   Ingrowing nail of the big toe. (Reproduced with permission from the Science Photo Library.)

Gout

Gout is an arthritis caused by the deposition of uric acid in the joint space, usually as a result of a metabolic failure to excrete this waste product. The first metatarsophalangeal joint is involved – **refer**.

Ingrowing toenail

Tight-fitting shoes and the temptation to cut the toenail too short (or with rounded rather than square edges) can result in the nail edge turning into the nail fold (Figure 15.5). The toe will be swollen and painful and may become infected. If unchecked, the nail bed granulates, producing a lump of fleshy tissue around and over the nail – **refer**.

Metatarsalgia

Metatarsalgia produces pain on weight bearing across the ball of the foot. It is a somewhat vague term applied to a variety of conditions. Chronic strain of the ligaments supporting the forefoot, with consequent loss of the lateral arch, is the most common explanation. It may be treated with rest, analgesia or anti-inflammatory drugs; if severe – **refer**.

Plantar fasciitis

The plantar fascia comprises two arch ligaments and a band of fibrous tissue overlying them and runs over the calcaneum (heel bone) to the toes. Plantar fasciitis is a chronic strain of the posterior attachment of the longitudinal arch ligament at its insertion into the calcaneum. It is also known as policeman's heel, a reference to the time when policemen were on their feet all day. The condition may be relieved by rest, but often recurs and requires treatment – **refer**.

Thrombosis

Occlusion of the arterial system can happen acutely or gradually. The usual clinical picture affects the elderly. There is a history of increasing vascular insufficiency with claudication and cold extremities. The acute episode is of sudden severe and constant pain, the foot and lower leg becoming white and pulseless. It is a medical emergency – **refer**.

(continued overleaf)

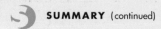 **SUMMARY** (continued)

Venous thrombosis affects a wider age range. It may particularly be suspected in younger patients taking oral contraceptives, and postoperatively, although both these are infrequent causes, with the move to low-dose oestrogens and the use of surgical anticoagulation. Again, the foot and (often) calf are painful, with oedema and in very severe cases a blue venous congestion of the skin – **refer**.

Verrucae

Verrucae are viral infections caused by the wart virus (the human papilloma virus). Usually affecting pressure areas of the foot, the lesion is constantly pushed into the epidermis, giving rise to the typical hard plaque of dry skin, with a small central ulcer revealing several black roots, which are in fact blood vessels (Figure 15.6). Verrucae may be treated with topical applications, or attempts can be made to destroy them with local cautery or freezing with liquid nitrogen.

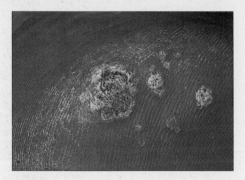

Figure 15.6   Verrucae. (Reproduced with permission from the Wellcome Trust Medical Photographic Library.)

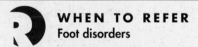 **WHEN TO REFER**
Foot disorders

- All diabetic patients with foot problems (refer to either the doctor or the chiropodist)

Refer to the chiropodist
- Bunions
- Calluses
- Corns
- Ingrowing toenail

Refer to the doctor
- Pain on weight bearing
- Severe sudden pain, with or without obvious inflammation in the first metatarsophalangeal joint of the big toe
- Foot colour and appearance abnormal, e.g. cold and white, swollen and blue/black (unless a healing sprain)
- Severe and lasting pain of sudden onset with no apparent cause such as trauma – urgent referral

CASE STUDIES

Case 1

A young man has made several visits to the pharmacy, usually buying fashionable and 'sporty' cosmetics, as well as antiperspirants and powders. On one occasion he also includes a prescription for emulsifying ointment and a moderately potent topical steroid. He sometimes has eczema, which he attributes to irritants from his job as a motor mechanic.

The pharmacist counsels him on the wisdom of the other things he is using on a potentially sensitised skin. He is a keen sportsman, mostly long distance running, which is often followed by socialising where he does not want the effects of his exertions to be apparent. He mentions that one thing that never leaves him is his smelly feet. He changes from running shoes immediately after exercise, but the irritation is not only embarrassing but often frankly painful.

The offending extremities are examined. The skin between three toes on both sides is red and dry, and very irritant. This erythema has spread onto the upper surface of the toes and encroaches on the dorsal surface of the feet. The diagnosis, appropriately enough, is athlete's foot (tinea pedis), aggravating adjoining eczema. Explanations are made and a treatment regime put in place. He will use clotrimazole and hydrocortisone cream between the toes night and morning for two to three weeks, and his emulsifying ointment on the remainder similarly for a few days, then once a day thereafter. The prescribed steroid cream is to be kept well out of the way.

The man is particularly keen not to stop training, with which the pharmacist has reservations, but about three weeks later he returns on an errand for his girlfriend sporting firstly the local half marathon medal and secondly an acceptance to the London full marathon.

'Personally', suggests the pharmacist wryly, 'I'd have stuck with the tinea.'

Case 2

A man in his mid 40s has an unusual request. While on holiday abroad he developed quite severe pain in his foot, and needed to see a local doctor. He is now on treatment, is improving but wonders whether the pharmacist can decipher the treatment he is taking and throw any light on the problem. The instructions on the two containers include much the pharmacist is unable to help with, but the list of ingredients mentions diclofenac and allopurinol. Gout is clearly the link, and this is discussed. The man remarks he thought he was rather young for this and is dismayed by the prospect of long-term therapy, but agrees that at least he is responding well to it.

The man returns a week later. The pain is worse again. Perhaps translation skills have been overestimated. On questioning, the NSAID, designed for short-term relief and to preserve his holiday, has finished, although the allopurinol continues. It just does not seem to work any more. The pharmacist enquires more closely. The pain did start around the head of the first metatarsal, but is now more widespread, along the full width of the 'ball' of the foot. He is advised to consult his doctor.

In a further week the man returns again, with a prescription for the anti-inflammatory alone. The doctor suggests metatarsalgia, and has asked for a further serum uric acid measurement, the result of which was not available by the end of the holiday. The doctor commented on the danger of assuming every pain in the great toe to be gout, and added that while his patient was taking a rich diet and more wine than his usual habit, he was also mountain walking.

'You probably don't do a lot of that round here.' he remarked.

The pharmacist agrees the diagnosis can be difficult, but refrains from mentioning it was a medical colleague that made it.

(continued overleaf)

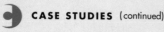 **CASE STUDIES** (continued)

Case 3

A man in his mid 60s calls in to pick up his usual medication and asks if he can buy some more of the verruca gel he has been using. The pharmacist cannot recall this and it transpires his daughter has been collecting it for him on her way home from work. Verrucae are uncommon in this age group and the pharmacist asks to see the foot. The heel is painful, the sole of the foot itching, with hyperkeratotic skin. As he does not wish to trouble the surgery, he is asked to leave off all treatment for a week or so, and then to be re-examined.

On re-examination there is still a hard tender pad of hyperkeratosis over the heel, with dry flaking skin on the sole, fissured along the sides, but no discrete lesion suggesting a verruca. It seems the gel may have been aggravating rather than improving matters. Emulsifying ointment is recommended at least twice a day, and every few days a soak in warm water with some of the ointment added. As the condition is more noticeable on one foot, a suggestion of ill-fitting shoes is tentatively made as the cause. Finally, the pharmacist concludes that should this regime fail then the doctor should be troubled, as other conditions such as psoriasis require consideration.

16

Oral and dental disorders

Guest contributor: Robin A Seymour BDS, PhD, FDSRC(Ed.)

Oral and dental disorders can be categorised into those affecting the teeth and the supporting structures (i.e. the gums and periodontal tissues; Figure 16.1) and disorders of the oral mucosa and associated structures (e.g. the lips, tongue, salivary glands and temporomandibular joint). The mouth is also often the site of adverse drug reactions and manifestations of systemic disease.

Assessing symptoms

The tooth

The most common dental complaint presenting to pharmacists is toothache. The patient will typically complain of continuous pain, usually of a throbbing nature. The pain may be exacerbated by hot, cold or sweet foods or drinks. Some patients have difficulty discerning which tooth is causing the pain. In many instances there may be an obviously carious or broken down tooth. Toothache may also arise as a result of a lost restoration (filling), from a heavily or recently restored tooth.

Pain arising when hot, cold or sweet stimuli are applied to the teeth may be due to dentine sensitivity arising as a consequence of gingival recession. This is invariably a localised sharp pain of short duration. Examination of the teeth will often show an area of gingival recession and exposed dentine.

Severe continuous pain may be caused by a dental abscess, which often arises from an infection of a necrotic dental pulp. Pain is often accompanied by localised swelling that can spread to parts of the face. The tooth is often slightly extruded from the socket. The commonest cause of pulpal necrosis is dental caries, although trauma and periodontal disease can compromise a tooth's vitality (i.e. its nerve and blood supply).

Pericoronitis is a specific infection arising in the soft tissue covering impacted third molars (wisdom teeth; Figure 16.2). Since these teeth erupt between the ages of 18 and 25 years, such infections are often seen in young adults. The infection is nearly always associated with lower third molars. A localised soreness in the soft

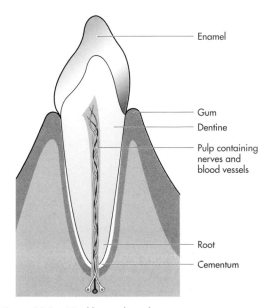

Figure 16.1 Healthy tooth and supporting structures.

Enamel

Gum

Dentine

Pulp containing nerves and blood vessels

Root

Cementum

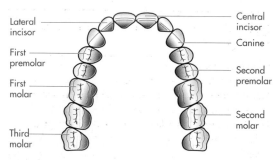

Figure 16.2   Permanent dentition of the upper dental arch.

tissues overlying an impacted or erupting tooth will develop into pain and swelling if untreated. Swelling is often buccal and, as with dental abscesses, can spread and potentially compromise the airway. It is very rare for pericoronitis to affect both lower third molars at the same time.

A localised continuous pain arising in a tooth socket some three to four days after tooth extraction may be due to a dry socket (alveolar osteitis). The precise cause is uncertain, but fibrinolysis of the blood clot appears to be important in the pathogenesis. The socket will be tender, show signs of breakdown of blood clots and poor healing, and there may be exposure of bone. Referral to a dental surgeon is necessary since the socket will require a dressing.

Supporting dental structures

The periodontal tissues are the supporting structures of the tooth in alveolar bone. They comprise gingiva (gums), periodontal ligament, root surface cementum and the lamina dura of the alveolar bone. Periodontal diseases are caused by bacterial plaque and compromise the supporting structures. Essentially these diseases can be classified into gingivitis, where plaque-induced inflammatory changes are confined to the gingival tissues, and periodontitis, where these changes have involved periodontal ligament and alveolar bone. Gingivitis is reversible whereas periodontitis is not, and treatment is aimed at preventing further loss of tissue.

Bleeding gums, especially on toothbrushing, is the most common symptom of gingivitis (see Figure 16.3). The patient may also complain of swelling and soreness of gums, particularly in the interdental area, and bad breath (halitosis). Plaque-induced gingival inflammatory changes can be exacerbated during pregnancy and at puberty.

Periodontitis is characterised by loss of periodontal attachment and resorption of alveolar bone. The condition is chronic and many patients are unaware that they have anything wrong with their teeth. The loss of supporting structures can result in gingival recession, pocket formation and an increase in tooth mobility. In advanced forms of periodontitis the teeth may become very loose and drop out. As with gingivitis, the causative agent is bacterial plaque.

A localised swelling adjacent to a tooth may be a periodontal abscess. Such an abscess is often chronic in nature and discharges pus in the mouth. Most periodontal abscesses are caused by Gram-negative micro-organisms. Occasionally they may be due to a foreign body lodged between the tooth and the gum.

A specific infection of the gingival tissues is acute necrotising ulcerative gingivitis (ANUG). In this condition there is pain, swelling and ulceration of the gingival tissues, particularly in the interproximal area.

Gingival overgrowth is a well-documented, unwanted effect associated with phenytoin, cyclosporin and calcium antagonists, particularly nifedipine. The prevalence of gingival over-

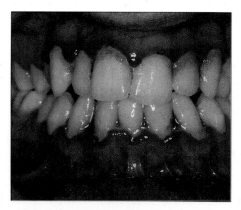

Figure 16.3   Gingivitis. (Reproduced with permission from the Newcastle Dental School.)

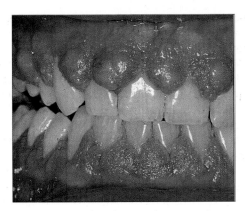

Figure 16.4 Drug-induced gingival overgrowth.
(Reproduced with permission from the Newcastle Dental School.)

Table 16.1   Drugs commonly implicated as causing xerostomia

Amphetamines
Antineoplastic drugs (occasionally)
Antiparkinson drugs, e.g. benzhexol (trihexyphenidyl),
    benztropine, orphenadrine
Antihistamines (H_1 blockers), atropine and atropine-
    like antispasmodics
Clonidine
Levodopa
Phenothiazines
Tricyclic and tetracyclic antidepressants

growth varies from drug to drug. For phenytoin, approximately 50 per cent of dentate patients are affected; this figure decreases to 30 per cent for cyclosporin and 10 per cent for nifedipine. Drug-induced gingival overgrowth (Figure 16.4) impedes mechanical plaque removal and the subsequent gingival inflammation further distorts the tissue.

Herpetic infections in the mouth are of two types: primary acute herpetic gingivostomatitis and herpes labialis (cold sore). The initial herpetic infection often occurs in children and can be confused with teething. The child is unwell, pyrexic and irritable. The gingival tissues are usually fiery red and very painful; vesicles may be present throughout the mouth, but these will usually have burst, leaving ulcerated areas. Acute herpetic gingivostomatitis is usually self-limiting, but the viral infection can recur in the form of cold sores. These usually start as a vesicle on the surface of the lips. The vesicle bursts and the raw area becomes crusted over. Healing occurs within seven to 10 days. Cold sores can be precipitated by trauma to the lips or sunlight. They tend to occur when patients are run down or suffering from other viral infections.

Oral mucosa

Dry mouth (xerostomia) can have a variety of causes, including mechnical obstruction of the salivary gland, drug therapy (Table 16.1) and Sjögren's syndrome. Sjögren's syndrome is a connective tissue disease of unknown aetiology. Features include dry mouth, dry eyes and rheumatoid arthritis.

A dry mouth is more prone to candidal infections and the reduced salivary flow increases the patient's susceptibility to caries, especially if there is gum recession causing exposure of the root surface. Apart from dryness of the mouth, patients with xerostomia will complain of difficulties in eating, swallowing and talking.

Aphthous ulceration of the oral mucosa is a troublesome, often recurrent problem that affects a large proportion of the population. Ulcers can occur in small crops, usually on the tongue, floor of the mouth or the base of the buccal fold (Figure 16.5). Once there is a break in the continuity of the epithelium the site becomes readily infected from the oral bacterial flora. Such infections delay ulcer healing. Some patients experience a burning or tingling sensation in

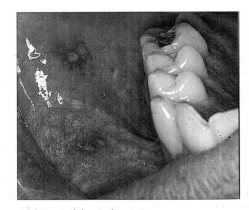

Figure 16.5 Aphthous ulceration. (Reproduced with permission from the Newcastle Dental School.)

certain parts of their mouth just before an outbreak of ulceration. Most patients tend to respond well to topical medication. The aetiology of aphthous ulceration is uncertain, but may be related to diet, hormonal changes, blood disorders or other causes.

Patients suffering from aphthous ulceration will complain of soreness of the mouth which is exacerbated by foods (especially spicy food). Ulcers often appear covered with a yellowish slough. They heal in seven to 10 days.

Lichen planus is a dermatological disorder that frequently involves the oral mucosa (Figure 16.6). Patients will complain of a sore mouth which is exacerbated by strong or spicy foods. The oral mucosa and gingival tissues are often ulcerated and show characteristic white striae (Wickham's striae).

Common candidal infections include thrush, denture-induced stomatitis and angular cheilitis. Such infections are characterised by a soreness of the mouth (Figure 16.7), a bad taste and discomfort on eating. This last problem is particularly likely if the patient wears dentures.

Candida albicans is an opportunistic commensal of the oral flora. Thrush infections are more common in babies and may be related to systemic antimicrobial therapy. Other types of *Candida* infections are frequently seen in edentulous elderly people wearing ill-fitting dentures. This so-called denture stomatitis is characterised by a fiery red palatal mucosa, which can exhibit hyperplasia. If there has been excessive wear on the dentures the patient becomes 'overclosed',

i.e. the dentures do not provide sufficient support for the facial tissues. This exacerbates the creases at the angles of the mouth which become infected with both candida and staphylococci (angular cheilitis). All candidal infections cause soreness of the oral mucosa. There is a tendency for the inflamed mucosa to bleed.

Lips

Cheilitis (inflammation of the lips; Figure 16.8) may be secondary to xerostomia, related to a systemic disease or caused by trauma or a hypersensitivity reaction. Symptoms can be of sudden onset and apart from being disfiguring, cheilitis will be associated with pain, soreness and problems with both eating and speech.

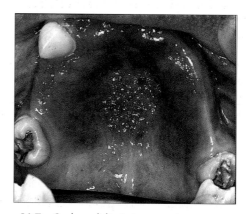

Figure 16.7   Oral candidiasis. (Reproduced with permission from the Newcastle Dental School.)

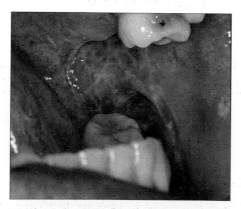

Figure 16.6   Erosive lichen planus. (Reproduced with permission from the Newcastle Dental School.)

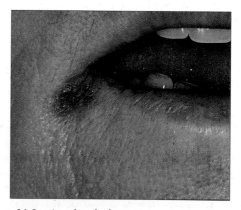

Figure 16.8   Angular cheilitis. (Reproduced with permission from the Newcastle Dental School.)

Tongue

Glossitis (inflammation of the tongue) can be caused by obvious pathology, such as ulceration or trauma, but in many cases it is difficult to establish a cause for the symptom. Iron and vitamin deficiencies (B_{12} and folate) are associated with glossitis but haematological screening often reveals no abnormality. Glossitis is often associated with burning mouth syndrome. In some cases allergic reactions to denture materials may be implicated.

A black hairy tongue is due primarily to a change in the tongue surface, notably an elongation of the filiform papillae, which is associated with the overgrowth of pigment-producing bacteria and fungi. The latter probably arises as a consequence of a disturbance in the normal oral flora. Drugs are the main cause of black hairy tongue, and those commonly implicated include penicillin and tetracyclines. The condition has also arisen following the use of oxygenation mouthwashes, such as those containing sodium perborate or hydrogen peroxide.

Black hairy tongue should be distinguished from black staining of the tongue, which can follow use of certain iron preparations.

Accompanying symptoms

Facial swelling may arise from a dental abscess, often with discharge of pus into the mouth, and should be regarded as serious, requiring referral to a doctor or dentist. Swelling in the soft tissue overlying an impacted or erupting third molar may be accompanied by difficulty in opening the mouth (trismus). The swelling is often buccal and potentially can compromise the airway. It requires referral.

A haemorrhage following a tooth extraction can arise within a few hours or two to three days after extraction. It is necessary to take a detailed history to ascertain whether there is any underlying cause, e.g. recent aspirin consumption, patient taking anticoagulant drugs or a haemorrhagic disorder. Early post-extraction haemorrhages are often due to a tear in the overlying gum (mucoperiosteum) and hence require suturing. Haemorrhage occurring two to three days

Table 16.2 Drugs commonly implicated as causing disturbances of taste

Aspirin	Imipramine
Carbimazole	Lithium carbonate
Chlorhexidine	Lincomycin
Clofibrate	Levodopa
Ethambutol	Metformin
Griseofulvin	Metronidazole
Gold salts	Penicillamine

after extraction is invariably due to infection and this requires appropriate treatment.

An unpleasant taste in the mouth and bad breath may accompany a dry socket or gingivitis. A foul halitosis is also often associated with ANUG. Taste disturbances may also be associated with a dry mouth. Some drugs cause taste disturbances (Table 16.2).

Onset and trigger factors

The pain of toothache and that associated with dentine sensitivity resulting from gingival recession is invariably exacerbated by hot, cold or sweet stimuli. Sensitivity to hot and cold stimuli can also arise in restored (filled) teeth. The latter may be due to a leaky (defective) filling that is poorly adapted to the tooth or to a lack of an insulating lining under the filling.

The pain of aphthous ulceration is stimulated by foods (especially spicy foods).

Pain arising three to four days after a tooth extraction may be due to a localised infection in the socket (dry socket or alveolar osteitis).

Gingival changes due to drugs can start within three months of commencing therapy; the gums of the upper and lower anterior teeth seem to be most affected (see Figure 16.4).

Special cases

Children

Teething is a common disorder associated with the eruption of the primary dentition. It is characterised by a localised inflammation of the gum overlying the erupting tooth and is associated with an increase in daytime restlessness, finger sucking, gum rubbing and drooling, sometimes with a temporary loss of appetite. Localised eruption cysts can occur during teething but these burst of their own accord. There is conflict as to whether teething produces any systemic disturbance. The child may be pyrexic, suffer from diarrhoea and be prone to upper respiratory tract infections while teething. Whether there is a link between tooth eruption and these constitutional disturbances has not been established.

Management

Tooth problems

Temporary fillings

A lost filling or other restoration (e.g. a crown) requires dental treatment for replacement. Temporary filling kits are available. These contain zinc oxide and eugenol, which the patient mixes to a thick paste and places into the cavity. A weaker mixture can be used to recement crowns – purely for cosmetic purposes. However, the emphasis must be placed on the temporary nature of the restorations provided by these kits. They are no substitute for appropriate treatment from a dental practitioner, but are useful in an emergency.

Dentine sensitivity

A variety of proprietary toothpastes contain active agents to reduce dentine sensitivity. These agents work by blocking the permeability of dentine to stimuli such as heat, cold and sweetness. Desensitising agents include strontium chloride, formaldehyde and stannous and sodium fluoride. The last two agents are also useful for preventing dental decay on exposed root surfaces. Toothpaste containing a desensitising agent should be used on a regular basis and relief occurs gradually over a period of several days. Excessive dentine sensitivity may be indicative of caries and therefore the patient should be advised to seek dental treatment.

Toothache

There is little effective treatment for toothache apart from extraction or filling (sometimes involving removal of the tooth pulp). Analgesics appear to afford little or no pain relief and the so-called toothache tinctures can cause burns to the gums. Furthermore, there is little evidence to suggest that such solutions actually relieve toothache.

Some patients believe that an aspirin tablet placed against the gum of the offending tooth will provide pain relief. This action will cause an aspirin burn on the oral mucosa and the patient should be warned accordingly. As with most dental disorders, the patient should be encouraged to seek dental treatment.

Dental abscesses require drainage and appropriate antibiotic therapy. If there is a discharge of pus, the patient should be advised to use a hot saline mouthrinse (e.g. one teaspoonful of salt in a cupful of water) to encourage further drainage. Severe infections should be referred to the casualty department of a hospital.

Pericoronitis likewise often requires antibiotic therapy and subsequent removal of the impacted tooth. Hot saline mouthrinses are of some value in reducing swelling, and simple OTC analgesics may afford some degree of pain relief.

Teething

There are many proprietary teething gels available as OTC products. Their active ingredient is usually a local anaesthetic agent (often lignocaine hydrochloride (lidocaine hydrochloride)) or an anti-inflammatory drug (e.g. choline salicylate). Although both types of product are claimed to reduce the local symptoms of teething, there is little clinical evidence to substantiate their use. Teething is often accompanied by pyrexia and paracetamol elixir (sugar free) should be recommended.

If teething is accompanied by diarrhoea, the child must be encouraged to take plenty of fluids.

Post-extraction conditions

Some post-extraction haemorrhages respond to simple pressure, achieved by the patient biting onto a clean pad of gauze. If this does not arrest haemorrhage, the patient should be referred back to the dental practitioner or to a casualty department since the socket will need packing and suturing.

Dry socket (alveolar osteitis) responds to local irrigation and the application of a proprietary dressing. Examples include bismuth iodoform paste, Whitehead's varnish impregnated into ribbon gauze, or a proprietary preparation containing butyl-paraminobenzoate (a topical anaesthetic), iodoform (an antiseptic) and eugenol, which provides further pain relief. Such local medicaments can only be applied by a dental practitioner. Occasionally, the patient may require a systemic antibiotic. There is little evidence that OTC painkillers are of any value in this condition.

Periodontal disorders

Periodontal disease is caused by the accumulation of bacterial plaque at the margin between tooth and gum and in between teeth. Most plaque can be removed by mechanical means using an appropriate tooth-brushing technique, interproximal cleaning aids and dental floss. However, many patients lack the motivation and dexterity to obtain zero or low plaque levels. It is against this background that there has been a considerable expansion in the development of agents to control plaque and periodontal disease.

Gingivitis is the early stages of periodontal disease and results from poor oral hygiene. Poor plaque control may have caused the problem and this needs to be rectified. However, since the gums are inflamed and bleed readily (see Figure 16.2), patients may be reluctant to clean their teeth thoroughly, especially with a new toothbrush. For these patients, a plaque-inhibitory agent (usually an antiseptic) may be of benefit. Many commercial plaque-inhibitory agents are available either as a mouthrinse or incorporated into toothpaste. Of the mouthrinses, chlorhexidine and those containing phenolic mixtures appear to be the most efficacious. These agents will only destroy or inhibit the formation of supragingival plaque and should be used in conjunction with mechanical plaque removal.

There are a variety of commercially available pre-brushing rinses which facilitate plaque removal by mechanical means. There is little evidence to support the efficacy of these agents in reducing gingival inflammation, and their regular use will not resolve bleeding and inflamed gums.

More advanced periodontal disease is characterised by movement of the teeth and an increased propensity to periodontal abscess formation. This condition requires specialised dental treatment and patients should be referred accordingly.

It is helpful if pharmacists stock a full range of oral hygiene aids to enable patients to optimise their plaque control programme.

Electric toothbrushes are of value where there is a problem handling a conventional toothbrush in patients with rheumatoid arthritis or other musculoskeletal disorders. Interproximal cleaning aids, e.g. brushes, wood sticks and various types of floss are of value.

It is thought that anaerobic bacteria play a significant role in the pathogenesis of ANUG. Most cases require referral for antimicrobial therapy, and metronidazole is the drug of choice. Early and mild cases of ANUG may respond to an oxygen-releasing mouthwash (e.g. sodium perborate).

Pharmacists should be aware of drugs that cause gingival overgrowth, if just to reassure the patient. Excessive gingival overgrowth is treated by surgical means, but in many patients the recurrence rate is high. If an alternative medication exists, it may be worthwhile contacting the patient's doctor to consider such a change. This policy may be particularly relevant for those patients who undergo repeated surgical procedures to correct their gingival overgrowth.

Disease of the oral mucosa

Dry mouth in the dentate patient will cause an increased susceptibility to dental caries. Fluoride mouthrinses will reduce this problem and these may be recommended. Salivary substitutes will certainly reduce (albeit temporarily) some oral discomfort associated with xerostomia. Preparations that are currently available are based on mucin, methylcellulose or carboxymethylcellulose. Various proprietary brands are available as aerosol sprays or pastilles. Dentate patients suffering from xerostomia may also obtain some relief by chewing sugar-free chewing gum.

For the edentulous patient, xerostomia poses the additional problem of poor dental retention. Denture fixative will be helpful to such patients. Salivary substitutes are also useful for these patients, together with lemon and glycerine pastilles or mouthwashes. These pastilles are unsuitable for dentate patients since the low pH value will increase the risk of dental caries. Patients with xerostomia are more prone to candidal infections, which should be treated with an appropriate antifungal agent (see below).

All patients with a history of recurrent aphthous ulceration require a full blood screening. The ulceration may be due to deficiencies in iron, vitamin B_{12} or folate. Symptomatic relief can be obtained with chlorhexidine mouthrinses (0.2 per cent w/v) or topical corticosteroids. Chlorhexidine reduces the incidence of secondary infection, which occurs shortly after the ulcer has formed. Topical corticosteroids in the form of pellets (hydrocortisone) and dental paste (triamcinolone) are available OTC. Some patients experience a burning sensation in their oral mucosa just prior to the outbreak of an ulcer. In these situations, local application of a corticosteroid can abort the outbreak.

Lip conditions

Acyclovir is the treatment of choice for herpetic infections. For primary herpetic gingivostomatitis referral for oral acyclovir is necessary. Herpes labialis (cold sores) should be treated with acyclovir cream 5 per cent, applied four to five times a day starting at the tingling phase, i.e. as early as possible. If sunlight is a causative factor in herpes labialis, the patient should be prescribed a sun block cream.

Treatment of cheilitis is often unsatisfactory and is dependent on the underlying cause. A lip salve will prevent further drying of the lips and this should be applied regularly. If the cheilitis is thought to be due to a hypersensitivity reaction, then a topical antihistamine cream may help to reduce symptoms.

Mouth disorders

The aetiology of glossitis and burning mouth syndrome is often multifactorial. This condition can be associated with vitamin B complex deficiency, hypersensitivity to denture materials, haematological deficiency, diabetes mellitus, reduced salivary function or psychological factors. Vitamin B therapy may be of some value, together with the use of salivary substitutes. It is obvious that these patients need a thorough appraisal to ascertain the cause of their symptoms.

Lichen planus requires treatment with topical corticosteroids (see aphthous ulceration) and severe cases may require systemic corticosteroids. If the lesions involve the gingival tissues, this will impede mechanical plaque removal. Regular use of a plaque-inhibitory agent such as chlorhexidine will help to alleviate this problem.

Candidiasis is the most frequent fungal infection affecting the oral mucosa. If the patient is dentate, an antifungal oral gel may be tried. Severe candidal infections require systemic antifungal agents. In edentulous patients, the fungal infection is often confined to the fitting area of the denture. For these patients, the denture should be thoroughly cleaned with a 1 per cent sodium hypochlorite solution at night and miconazole gel applied to the fitting surface of the denture four times a day.

Angular cheilitis (see Figure 16.8) is often caused by both *Candida* and *Staphylococcus aureus*. Miconazole gel is the treatment of choice for this condition since it possesses both antimycotic and antibacterial properties.

There is no treatment of black hairy tongue apart from reassurance. The condition will usually resolve on cessation of any causative drugs. Brushing the tongue with a toothbrush may help to disperse the pigment-producing bacteria and reduce the length of the filiform papillae.

Staining and discoloration of the teeth

There are many causes for staining or discoloration of the teeth, ranging from rare genetic defects in tooth formation, dental caries, excessive intake of fluoride (fluorosis) and dietary factors. Simple extrinsic staining arising from smoking, excessive coffee intake or chewing betel nut can be removed in part by short-term use of an abrasive toothpaste. Resistant stains need professional cleaning.

Defects in the tooth surface will require repair and coverage with a veneer. Similarly, tetracycline staining of the teeth can be covered using thin porcelain veneers.

Prevention of dental caries

Over the past 20 years, there has been a significant decline in the prevalence of dental caries. Fluoride has been mainly responsible for this decline, either through the water supply or its incorporation into toothpastes. In spite of these measures, there is still a need for further action to maintain the decline in dental caries.

Dietary advice is paramount in any caries prevention programme. Particular attention should focus on the intake of refined carbohydrates and snacking between meals. Confectionery taken between meals causes a significant drop in the pH of the oral environment, rendering the teeth more prone to acid attack. Chewing gum stimulates salivary flow, which buffers the oral environment to this acid attack and helps promote remineralisation of the tooth surface.

Fissure sealants applied professionally do reduce the incidence of dental caries on the occlusal (biting) surface of posterior teeth. However, such sealants should not be an excuse for over-indulgence in confectionery or avoidance of regular tooth-brushing. It is important for the maintenance of oral health that these measures are attended to.

Bacterial plaque is the main aetiological agent in dental caries. Regular tooth-brushing (at least twice/day) will remove most plaque deposits and hence reduce the bacterial challenge on the tooth surfaces.

SUMMARY OF ORAL AND DENTAL DISORDERS

Lost filling or other restoration
Fillings and other restorations can be lost following fracture of a tooth cusp secondary to recurrent dental caries or, in the case of a crown or a bridge, fracture of the dental cement. Eating sticky foods such as toffee can readily displace a restoration – **refer**.

Sensitivity of the teeth
Sensitivity arises as a result of either gingival recession or periodontal disease. The exposed root surface is sensitive to hot, cold or sweet stimuli, which produce pain, often of a short, sharp nature. Dentine sensitivity responds to toothpastes that contain active agents such as sodium fluoride, strontium chloride or formaldehyde. Intractable cases may require a permanent restoration.

Teething
Soreness of the gums often accompanies the eruption of the primary dentition. Local application of gels containing lignocaine (lidocaine) or choline salicylate may afford relief until the tooth erupts through the mucosa. Teething is often associated with pyrexia, for which paracetamol elixir is recommended.
(continued overleaf)

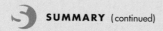 **SUMMARY** (continued)

Dental abscess

Dental abscesses are often due to a necrotic dental pulp. They can present as a localised swelling associated with the tooth or marked facial swelling. The latter requires urgent treatment with antibiotics and drainage – **refer**.

Pericoronitis

Pericoronitis is an infection associated with the eruption of third molars (wisdom teeth). It may present initially as a localised soreness over the erupting tooth, but can progress to cause severe facial swelling and restriction in mouth opening (trismus). Antimicrobials are the treatment of choice, followed by extraction of the third molar. Hot saline mouthwashes may provide some temporary relief in mild cases – **refer**.

Toothache

Toothache (pulpitis) can present as severe pain, often of a throbbing nature. Pain is exacerbated by hot and cold stimuli. The pain may be accompanied by abscess formation. Analgesics afford little or no relief – **refer**.

Post-extraction haemorrhage

Most post-extraction haemorrhages are caused by a tear in the gingival tissues. Some can be arrested by biting on gauze. If this fails, the patient requires the socket to be packed and sutured, hence – **refer**. It is important to check that the patient has no bleeding disorders and is not taking drugs that interfere with haemostasis.

Dry socket

Dry socket (alveolar osteitis) is a localised infection arising in the tooth socket some two to four days after tooth extraction. The pain is localised, continuous and can radiate along the jaws. Treatment involves debridement of the tooth socket, followed by the insertion of a local dressing. Antibiotics may be required in severe cases – **refer**.

Periodontal disorders

Periodontal diseases are caused by bacterial plaque. Gingivitis is the early manifestation of periodontal disease and is characterised by bleeding, sore gums (see Figure 16.2) and often bad breath. Treatment is aimed at improving oral hygiene with particular attention to toothbrushing and interproximal tooth cleaning. Plaque-inhibitory agents have a significant effect on bacterial plaque and help to resolve the inflammatory changes in the gingival tissues.

   More advanced periodontal disease (periodontitis) is characterised by loss of the supporting dental structures (the periodontium) and resorption of alveolar bone. The condition is chronic. It can result in gingival recession, movement and spacing of the teeth and an increase in tooth mobility. Local abscess formation can occur. Plaque-control measures are essential for the successful management of periodontitis, but such measures do not remove plaque from beneath the gingival margins – **refer**.

Acute necrotising ulcerative gingivitis

This is a condition of uncertain aetiology characterised by soreness and local ulceration of the gingival tissues. It is accompanied by a foul smell and may be localised to a few teeth or generalised. Poor oral hygiene, smoking and general debilitating illness (especially HIV infection) predispose patients to this infection. Mild cases may respond to a mouthrinse containing an oxygen-releasing agent. More established cases require antimicrobial therapy, hence – **refer**.

→

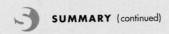

SUMMARY (continued)

Gingival overgrowth

This is an unwanted effect associated with phenytoin, cyclosporin and some calcium antagonists. Gingival overgrowth can be severe, disfiguring and interfere with both speech and eating (see Figure 16.4). Gingival changes also impede mechanical plaque removal, which exacerbates the condition. Drug-induced gingival overgrowth is treated by surgery but the recurrence rate is high. Alternative medication may be appropriate (if available) for those patients who experience recurrence of this unwanted effect. In such cases – **refer**.

Dry mouth

The causes of dry mouth (xerostomia) are many and varied, e.g. following radiotherapy to the head and neck, secondary to Sjögren's syndrome and drugs. The consequences include soreness of the oral mucosa, lips and tongue, difficulty in eating and speech, and an increased propensity to oral infections (especially candidiasis) and caries. Artificial salivas, sugar-free chewing gum and, for the edentulous patient, lemon and glycerine pastilles are useful.

Aphthous ulceration

Recurrent ulceration of the oral mucosa is a common condition causing localised soreness and pain (see Figure 16.5). Patients require thorough investigation to elucidate and treat any underlying cause. The ulcers occur in crops and in some patients their outbreak is preceded by a tingling/burning sensation in the oral mucosa. Local antiseptics, such as chlorhexidine, reduce the incidence and severity of secondary infection and promote healing. Topical corticosteroids are the treatment of choice; their efficacy is related to use as early as possible in the course of the ulceration. If severe or recurrent – **refer**.

Herpetic infections

Acute herpetic gingivostomatitis (AHGS) and herpes labialis are the two principal oral herpetic infections. AHGS is more likely to occur in children and is sometimes confused with teething. The condition is very painful and is characterised by vesicles on the tongue, gingiva and hard palate. These burst to leave ulcers, which readily become secondarily infected. The infection is often accompanied by pyrexia and lymphadenopathy. Patients will complain of marked pain and soreness of the mouth that is exacerbated by eating and swallowing – **refer**.

Cold sores are a recurrent form of herpetic infection which break out on the borders of the lips. A vesicle may form, which bursts to leave a small raw area. Acyclovir cream is the treatment of choice.

Glossitis and burning mouth

These two conditions often occur together and are difficult to treat. Patients need thorough investigation to identify any predisposing cause – **refer**.

Lichen planus

Lichen planus is a condition of unknown aetiology that is characterised by bouts of disease activity followed by periods of quiescence. Erosive, ulcerated lesions occur, usually on the gingival tissues and buccal mucosa (see Figure 16.6). Treatment involves topical and occasional systemic corticosteroids – **refer**.

(continued overleaf)

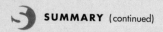

SUMMARY (continued)

Candidal infections
Candidal infections (see Figure 16.7) cause soreness of the mouth and occur more frequently at the extremes of age. They are particularly common among denture wearers. Treatment is with a topical anti-fungal gel in the first instance and this can also be applied to the fitting surface of the denture

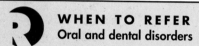

WHEN TO REFER
Oral and dental disorders

(Referral can be to either a doctor or a dentist)

Teeth and gums
- Continuous pain that does not improve
- Swelling of the gums
- Sharp pain of short duration, aggravated by hot or cold stimuli, that does not respond to treatment with a desensitising toothpaste
- Lost filling
- Soreness and pain over impacted third molars (wisdom teeth) in a young adult
- Post-extraction pain
- Bleeding or painful gums
- Gum recession, together with movement of the teeth within the socket

Oral mucosa and lips
- Persistently inflamed, sore or painful tongue
- White patches on the buccal mucosa or tongue
- Mouth ulcers that do not respond to OTC local steroid treatment
- Dry mouth

Other
- Facial swelling
- Trismus (limited mouth opening)
- Haemorrhage from a tooth socket
- Severe halitosis
- Taste disturbance
- Inflammation of the tongue
- Hairy black tongue

CASE STUDIES

Case 1

One of the pleasures of community pharmacy is helping mothers through early parenthood with advice and often with reassurance. Most problems are minor, although vigilance is always necessary.

A young woman well known to her pharmacist calls early one morning. Her child of six months has been teething again and they both have had a sleepless night. Could she have a further supply of the medication they have found so successful before? The pharmacist commiserates and notices that both mother and child seem more distressed and agitated than expected. Coming round the counter, the pharmacist finds the child pyrexial, with sores on the edge of her mouth. Closer inspection reveals her to be dribbling profusely with her gums fiery red. It seems likely that the child has a stomatitis, probably herpetic. The pharmacist explains that on this occasion the doctor should see the child, adding that there is nothing very serious and the doctor may well not prescribe for the condition. The mother and child leave, already more cheerful and the pharmacist is reminded that occasionally people need permission even to ask for advice.

The mother returns a week later for a repeat prescription of her contraceptive, apologetic that she did not report back earlier. The doctor concurred with the diagnosis, advised fluids, rest and paracetamol, and saw her daughter again three days later, when she was already recovering. She is very impressed with the pharmacist's diagnostic skills.

Case 2

A young man asks for a large pack of paracetamol, unless the pharmacist can recommend anything stronger. He is obviously in considerable pain, holding one side of his face and having difficulty speaking. There is a noticeable swelling and he has felt feverish. Also he has taken almost 20 paracetamol in the last 36 hours. The pharmacist is reluctant to supply either a further large quantity of paracetamol or a combination product, and advises he should seek an urgent dental opinion. The young man is hesitant, put off by the anticipated cost and the fact that he is very overdue to have a check up. The pharmacist explains that he probably has a dental infection, and if not treated promptly it may progress to an abscess and require draining, as well as threatening his teeth.

The advice is taken and the man returns the following morning with a prescription for amoxicillin. An old filling has been removed, the pressure relieved and the pain is subsiding.

Case 3

A young woman in her mid 20s asks the pharmacist to recommend something for her sore mouth. She has been advised it could be cold sores, and she is embarrassed to think she might pass them on to other people.

On closer questioning it is found that she has no sores around her lips, instead they take the form of ulcers on her tongue and the floor of her mouth, and although she has nothing to show at the moment, the probable diagnosis is aphthous ulceration. The pharmacist is happy to make a recommendation, although would have preferred to see a lesion first to confirm.

This is not a problem, she replies, as they always occur premenstrually, and can be predicted.

(continued overleaf)

CASE STUDIES (continued)

'Like so many things around that time,' she adds.

Perhaps the pharmacist might like to include something for her headaches, fluid retention and heavy periods as well.

The pattern thus emerges of a whole range of hormonally related problems. Medication is recommended for her mouth ulcers, as the next period is imminent, as is a consultation with her doctor to review the broader symptoms. She is amused to think a change of her contraceptive pill might help mouth ulcers: the pharmacist reflects on how often one seemingly minor problem is part of a distant but more significant condition.

Index

Page numbers in *italics* refer to tables; those in **bold** to figures. The alphabetical arrangement is letter-by-letter.